Pre-eclampsia

Pre-eclampsia

Prevention, Prediction and Possibilities

Pankaj Desai

Dean (Students)
A. Professor and Unit Chief (VR)
Department of Obgyn, Medical College and S.S.G. Hospital
Vadodara, India

Consultant Obgyn Specialist
Janani Maternity Hospital
Vadodara, India

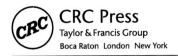

CRC Press
Taylor & Francis Group
Boca Raton London New York

CRC Press is an imprint of the
Taylor & Francis Group, an **informa** business

First edition published 2021
by CRC Press
6000 Broken Sound Parkway NW, Suite 300, Boca Raton, FL 33487-2742

and by CRC Press
2 Park Square, Milton Park, Abingdon, Oxon, OX14 4RN

ISBN: 9780367135072 (hbk)
ISBN: 9780367086046 (pbk)
ISBN: 9780429023286 (ebk)

Typeset in Minion
by Lumina Datamatics Limited

Contents

Preface   xi

Acknowledgements   xiii

Author   xv

PART 1   GENERAL ASPECTS OF PRE-ECLAMPSIA   1

1   **Introduction**   3
    General aspects of pre-eclampsia   3
    What is pre-eclampsia?   4
    What is obstetric vasculopathy?   4

PART 2   POSSIBILITIES IN AETIOLOGY OF PRE-ECLAMPSIA   7

2   **Immunology of pre-eclampsia**   9
    Immune tolerance and pre-eclampsia   9
    Types of pre-eclampsia based on immunology   9
    First few days of placentation and pre-eclampsia   10
    The autonomous tight unit   10
    Uterine glands and placentation   10
        Uterine milk   11
        Uterine gland knockout cells   11
        The crosstalk   12
    References   12
3   **Endothelial cell dysfunction and pre-eclampsia**   15
    Introduction   15
    The phenomenon of endothelial cell activation   16
    Circulating markers of endothelial activation   16
    Endothelial activation and prostaglandins   16
    Plasminogen and allied procoagulant activity: A manifestation of endothelial cell activation   17
    Antiphospholipid antibodies act through procoagulant mechanism   17
    Endothelial cell adhesion molecule disturbances   18
    VEGF   18
        Clinical bearings   18
    Endothelin   19

	Other molecules contributing to endothelial cell activation	19
	Immunological antibodies	19
	Cytokines	19
	Formed elements in blood	20
	"Toxins"	20
	List of Abbreviations	20
	References	20
4	**Oxidative stress and pre-eclampsia**	**23**
	Introduction	23
	What is oxidative stress?	23
	What is a free radical?	23
	Oxygen: A double-edged sword	24
	The mischief of free radicals in vascular walls	25
	Lipid peroxides: The agents of oxidative stress	25
	Our basic study	28
	Lipid metabolism in normal pregnancy and in pre-eclampsia	28
	Hypertriglyceridemia and pre-eclampsia	31
	Small dense LDL phenotype in pre-eclampsia	31
	Placental lipid peroxidation	32
	Transition metals in lipid peroxidation	34
	Clinical manifestations	35
	Reperfusion	35
	Innate maternal reducing systems	37
	The family of free radicals	38
	Vascular endothelium and oxidative stress	38
	Inefficient second wave of trophoblastic invasion	39
	Production of vascular endothelial growth factors	40
	Nitric oxide in pre-eclampsia	41
	Nitric oxide and endothelial cells	41
	Placental atherosis in pre-eclampsia	42
	Extracellular reducing systems	42
	Uric acid: The powerhouse reductant	43
	Policeman-to-riot model to understand uric acid	43
	Limitations of reducing systems	44
	Inconsistency of reducing systems	45
	The ideal reducing system	45
	Exercise and prevention of pre-eclampsia	45
	The beauty of lysophosphotidyl choline	46
	References	47
5	**Metabolic syndrome and pre-eclampsia**	**51**
	What is metabolic syndrome?	51
	Metabolic syndrome and hypertension	51
	Metabolic changes in normal pregnancy	52
	Basal metabolic rate	52
	Proteins and amino acids	53
	Carbohydrates	53
	Lipids	53
	Diagnosis of metabolic syndrome	54
	Metabolic syndrome and pre-eclampsia	54
	References	54

6   The genetics of pre-eclampsia   **57**
Basis for reviewing the role of genetics in pre-eclampsia   57
Challenges to the genetic studies in pre-eclampsia   58
Mammalian studies   59
Application of genetic models   59
Examining associations   59
Foetal contributions: Any?   59
Immunology and genetics   60
Epigenetics and pre-eclampsia   61
References   61

PART 3   PREDICTION   **63**

7   Prediction of pre-eclampsia   **65**
Introduction   65
Challenges to tests for prediction in pre-eclampsia   65
Need for multiple tests   65
Assessing the quality of tests in prediction of pre-eclampsia   65
Overview of the types of tests   66
Clinical bearings of negative and positive tests   66
An ideal test   66
Clinical tests   66
    Mid-trimester blood pressure   66
    The roll-over test   67
    Hand-grip test   67
    Maternal weight gain in pregnancy   67
Urinary tests   67
    Microalbuminuria   67
    Urinary calcium   68
    Calcium-to-creatinine ratio   68
    Kallikrein   68
Haematological indices   68
    Cellular components in prediction of pre-eclampsia   68
        Leucocytes   68
        Platelets and platelet activation   68
        Uric acid   69
        Fibronectin   70
        β-hCG   70
Epidemiological indices in pre-eclampsia prediction   70
Colour Doppler in pre-eclampsia prediction: The game changer   71
    Review of indices   71
    Doppler indices with biomarkers   72
    The diastolic notch   72
    What is diastolic notch?   72
    Practical problem with using colour Doppler and biomarker in combination   73
    Notch Depth Index   74
    Doppler indices for the discontinuation of preventive measures   75
    Identifying low-risk subjects in the first trimester   76
The future: Nanoparticles including exosomes   76
References   77

PART 4 PREVENTION   **81**

8   **Prevention of pre-eclampsia**   **83**
  Introduction   83
  What is the difference between disease and derangement?   83
  Which subjects may benefit?   85
  Salt restriction   85
  Diuretics   85
  Antihypertensives   86
  Calcium supplementation   86
  Other trace elements and micronutrients   87
  Aspirin for the prevention of pre-eclampsia   87
  Possible mechanism of action of aspirin   87
  Aspirin: Review of literature   88
  What dose of aspirin: 75 mg or 150 mg?   88
  Misgivings and fears about aspirin   89
  Aspirin timing   89
  References   89

PART 5 SYSTEMIC MANIFESTATIONS   **93**

9   **Central nervous system**   **95**
  Changes in the CNS   95
  Pathological lesions in pre-eclampsia   95
    Brain   96
  Posterior leukoencephalopathy syndrome   96
  Psychiatric complications following obstetric vasculopathies: Any correlation?   96
  References   96

10   **Cardiovascular system**   **99**
  Changes in cardiac functions   99
  Stroke volume and heart rate   99
  How does the heart increase its cardiac output?   99
  Vascular response to increase cardiac output   100
  Oscillatory pressure and propulsive pressure   100
  Peripheral vascular resistance   101
  Changes in venous system   101
  References   102

11   **Haematological system**   **103**
  Introduction   103
  Alteration in coagulation factors (other than platelets) and procoagulants   103
  Alteration in other cellular components of blood   103
  Review of coagulation alterations in pre-eclampsia   104
  Platelets in normal and pre-eclamptic pregnancies   104
  Concept of competence alteration (efficiency) of platelets   105
  Platelet activation and thromboxane A_2 production   105
  References   106

12   **Hepatobiliary system**   **109**
  Introduction   109
  Pathological changes in the liver   109
  Liver in the HELLP syndrome   110
  References   110

13   **Ophthalmic system**   **113**
      Introduction   113
      The peripheral pathogenesis of ophthalmic changes in pre-eclampsia   113
      The central pathogenesis of ophthalmic changes in pre-eclampsia   114
      Visual alterations of special mention – recurrent and unilateral   114
      References   114
14   **Renal system**   **117**
      Introduction   117
      Brief outline of renal changes in pregnancy   117
      Vulnerability of renal system   117
      Special features of renal failure complicating pre-eclampsia   118
      Renal lesions   119
      Are kidney changes in pre-eclampsia – pathognomonic?   119
      Gross changes in the kidneys   119
      On microscopy   119
      Renal function alterations in pre-eclampsia   121
      Renal handling of proteins in pre-eclampsia   122
          Handling of urinary excretion of proteins in pre-eclampsia   122
      Renin-angiotensin system in pre-eclampsia   122
      References   123

PART 6   CLINICAL FEATURES OF PRE-ECLAMPSIA   **125**

15   **Clinical features**   **127**
      Introduction   127
      Classification   127
      Hypertension   128
      Proteinuria   128
      Oedema   129
      Grades of severity of pre-eclampsia   129
      References   129

PART 7   TREATMENT OF PRE-ECLAMPSIA   **131**

16   **Treatment of pre-eclampsia**   **133**
      Introduction   133
      Management goals in pre-eclampsia   133
      Early diagnosis and alert surveillance   133
      Do women with pre-eclampsia need admission?   134
      Management on hospitalization   134
          Antihypertensives   135
              Does mild pre-eclampsia need antihypertensives?   135
              Challenges before treating pre-eclampsia with antihypertensives   135
              Which antihypertensive?   136
              Mono therapy versus multi-drug therapy   136
              Drugs and their dosage schedules   137
              When to stop antihypertensives   137
          Induction of labour in PIH   137
              37 weeks   138
              Induction of labour in eclampsia   138

Induction of labour in severe pre-eclampsia 138
Induction of labour in pregnancy for foetal reasons 138
Case study in CPR 139
Analysis of the case study 143
The need for involving a neonatologist 144
Readiness of the maternal system for labour induction in PIH 144
Methods of the induction of labour 144
Trachleodynamics in the induction of labour 144
Prostaglandins 145
Dose 145
Foley catheters in induction of labour 146
Other methods of labour induction 146
Caesarean section in PIH 146
Post-delivery care 147
Postpartum haemorrhage (PPH) 147
Blood pressure 147
Coagulation failure 147
Renal failure 148
Pulmonary oedema 148
References 148

Index **151**

Preface

Recurrent miscarriages fascinated me in my academic journey through obstetrics. This journey is nearly four decades old. Why should some pregnancies fail again and again when millions end successfully? This intrigue brought me to the doors of immunology of pregnancy. The complexity of why and how a pregnancy gets tolerated bound me to it. One thing led to another, and my forays into the entire larger concept of obstetric vasculopathies deepened. It was a continuous process of learning and discovering. Sometimes the attempts met with success, and other times ended in failure.

While the association of immunology and different obstetric vasculopathies was getting well established, interest in pre-eclampsia automatically resulted. Unclear aetiology, a myriad prediction tests and emerging competent prevention methods were those aspects of pre-eclampsia that proved to be most fascinating. One condition – pre-eclampsia and its two completely different characteristics – proved to be quite fascinating. The two characteristics are – pre-eclampsia remote from term (at or before 34 weeks of pregnancy) and late-onset pre-eclampsia. Pre-eclampsia remote from term, the most furious and scarier form of pre-eclampsia, has its origin at the foetomaternal interface, and pre-eclampsia of late onset has probably a non-placental origin. Both have the same clinical manifestations, but still their characteristics are completely different. At every turn, I was amazed. The role of uterine glands, the concept of uterine milk and what both do in causing obstetric vasculopathies in general and pre-eclampsia in particular were simply awesome intrigues of nature.

When one studies these conditions, it soon becomes obvious that the origin of pre-eclampsia cannot occur late in pregnancy. Pre-eclampsia must begin in the first few days after conception and implantation. The foetomaternal interface in the first trimester is completely autonomous. Even the mother has no control over it; this is necessary for a healthy obstetric outcome at term. In this autonomous system, the environment is essentially anaerobic – even an atom of oxygen is not allowed to seep in. So here on the outside is the mother who cannot survive without oxygen and on the other side, the developing foetus in the mother's body that cannot tolerate even micro amounts of oxygen. This may be necessary because this is the all-important phase of organogenesis.

In this tightly closed environment, one aspect that is cardinal is how the maternal decidual cells communicate with the foetal system. This communication has to be robust, competent and healthy. Exosomes are the communication tools whose roles are being increasingly studied in occurrences of pre-eclampsia. Originally found to have an important role in malignancy, exosomes are now being investigated for their role in pre-eclampsia. Standardisation of laboratory methods to assess exosomes can, in all likelihood, detail their role in the prediction of pre-eclampsia. Extending it further, stem cells can be used to manipulate these communication tools in such a way that the failure or ineffective crosstalk does not occur. This would subsequently lead to the prevention of pre-eclampsia most specifically and accurately. This is the future.

The amorphously understood aetiology leads to discoveries of different methods in predicting pre-eclampsia. Methods studied include clinical, biochemical and colour Doppler, which are all reviewed in this book. Also reviewed are methods in preventing pre-eclampsia – aspirin being the mainstay in this. Clinical features of and treatment methods for pre-eclampsia are covered extensively in the light of current literature.

The project of writing, rewriting and reviewing this book lasted longer than a year. But as the book took a solid shape, I felt a sense of satisfaction. All the painstaking efforts, the diligence and day-to-day work was all worth it. It was an exercise in revelations of different intrigues of nature, the complexities of pathological processes and derangements of the physiology of pregnancy. It has, at times, left me absolutely awestruck. Pre-eclampsia revealed so many of its forms – that of a loving mother or a ferocious foe or a tamed pet or a hidden mystery all rolled in one. The more one knows about pre-eclampsia, the more it tries to hide. This leaves the investigator absolutely humble and thirsty to know still more.

As I place this book in the hands of readers, I feel satisfied and blessed. I hope it proves to be one more step in my pursuit of scientific excellence at the service of humanity and humankind.

Acknowledgements

Someone has beautifully said "At times, our own light goes out and is rekindled by a spark from another person. Each of us has cause to think with deep gratitude of those who have lighted the flame within us". I felt this all throughout my experiences with pre-eclampsia and during this entire process of writing this book. I owe a profound thankfulness to my parents; my elder brother, Ganesh; my wife, Meera; my daughter, Ushma; and my son and daughter-in-law, Shlok and Prarthana for their support, encouragement and their warmth throughout the process of writing this book. I can never thank enough all those countless patients from whom I could fathom the amazing mysteries of pre-eclampsia. My special thanks to all my amazing students throughout my career as a teacher in medical college whom I had a great opportunity to teach and thereby, learn from. They were a great source of backing for me in my academic journey. The entire staff of Taylor & Francis Group that was involved in the process of making this book deserves a special thanks. I have three non-biological mothers: Rosary School, Medical College – Baroda and the Federation of Obstetric & Gynaecological Societies of India (FOGSI). Without these three in my life, I would be nothing. I have no words to thank these mothers of mine for entire role in making me and therefore, this book in its current form.

आवाहनं न जानामि न जानामि तवार्चनम।

पूजां चैव न जानामि क्षम्यतां परमेश्वरि।।

मंत्रहीनं क्रियाहीनं भक्तिहीनं सुरेश्वरि।

यत्पूजितं मया देवि परिपूर्णं तदस्तु मे।।

[I do not know the rites and rituals, I do not even know how to worship you. I cannot even make a proper appeal to you. Please forgive me for that. I can only love you. Please accept my love and incomplete efforts, with love.]

Author

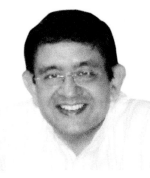

Dr. **Pankaj Desai** is one of the best-known academicians and teachers in obstetrics and gynaecology in India. All his 12 books have proved to be best-sellers, one of which was awarded the best book award in the subject. A prolific writer, he has contributed 43 chapters to different textbooks internationally and nationally. His outstanding academic contributions in the subject have been acknowledged and honoured with 7 gold medals and 60 orations. An extremely popular teacher, he has delivered 717 guest lectures in different parts of India and all over the world. He has published 107 research papers, 9 of which have been awarded best research paper prizes. His website www.drpankajdesai.com has become an extremely popular portal for students and practitioners of the subject seeking references and up-to-date knowledge of the subject; it has nearly 200,000 hits at the time of publication. His blogs on different academic and non-academic aspects, published as Dr. Pankaj Desai's blogs, have also become popular with more than 80,000 reads. He was recently felicitated by his large number of students and was called The Best Teacher of the Century!

PART 1

General aspects of pre-eclampsia

Introduction

GENERAL ASPECTS OF PRE-ECLAMPSIA

Of all systems in the human body, the reproductive system is probably the last on the priority list of nature. With any life-threatening crisis looming on the horizon, the first to be shut down is the reproductive system. As if by magic, it takes hardly any time for the process of physiology to get deranged and diseased. During the course of my journey through the science of obstetrics, adverse outcomes always intrigued me. Three questions have been the greatest drivers in all sciences. Right from the definition of time and space by Aristotle to his scientific investigations into the same by Isaac Newton and over to the astounding precepts by Albert Einstein, all progress in science has been driven by these three questions: Why? What if? and How? These questions permeate through all progress in science, including the most complex obstetric derangement of obstetric vasculopathies.

As a junior resident pursuing my post-MBBS studies in the labour ward, I once received two mothers with PIH one after another in quick succession. The first was a full-term pregnant woman, who had a blood pressure of 150/100 mmHg, had oedema and trace of albuminuria. The second subject had only a mid-trimester pregnancy of about 22 weeks, a blood pressure of 160/110 mmHg, oedema and very high albuminuria. The first subject went on to deliver vaginally a 2.9-kg child who was healthy and alive. The second woman with the same disease had to be induced because her blood pressure progressively got more dangerous. The baby could not be saved, and the mother took a long time to get her blood pressure back to a normal state. She stayed in the hospital for nearly 3 months. Many such patients came and went, and each time I got challenged, "Why did she have this outcome? Why not the others?"

As a couple of years rolled by, I saw these same mothers for subsequent obstetric services. In her next pregnancy, the first mother who had a milder form of the disease did not have PIH or any other high-risk factor. She delivered vaginally uneventfully and left. The second mother (who had a severe form of the disease and that early in pregnancy) came in at her next pregnancy, which resulted in a foetal demise at 10 weeks. Her third pregnancy in which I attended to her, she had an IUGR with accidental haemorrhage. Incidentally, she managed to reach 34 weeks, but she had to be sectioned out by a lower segment caesarean section (LSCS) and went home after nearly a month in the hospital. Her blood pressure had shot up nearing delivery, and it took nearly a month for it to reach a normal state again. Concurrently, her baby was admitted to the neonatal intensive care unit (NICU), but the silver lining was that this time, the pregnancy resulted in a live neonate.

Seemingly diverse obstetric conditions: severe PIH remote from term, IUGR, accidental haemorrhage and foetal demise all occurred in the same mother in different pregnancies. Are those interlinked conditions? If yes, in what way they are interlinked? What binds them together? Do they have some long-term effects? Above all, what causes them? How does one treat these conditions?

Those were the early years of the 1980s. The institution where I worked did not have any facilities for ultrasound or a colour Doppler then. Using aspirin was still scoffed at. We had just begun to use magnesium sulphate to treat eclampsia. There were no computers to manage the data, and at best, we had calculators to calculate statistical indices. Our first study on this matter titled, "Preeclampsia remote from term" was presented at the All India Conference of Obstetrics & Gynaecology at Jaipur. The study showed interesting results; and it was the harbinger of more than two decades of diligent and dedicated study of these conditions which are now known as "Obstetric Vasculopathies".

WHAT IS PRE-ECLAMPSIA?

Pre-eclampsia is a pregnancy complication characterised by high blood pressure and signs of damage to another organ system, most often the liver and kidneys. It may be accompanied by albuminuria or oedema. It usually begins after 20 weeks of pregnancy in women whose blood pressure has been normal. This is the standard definition of pre-eclampsia.

There have been many attempts to produce animal models that mimic the hypertensive disorders of pregnancy, especially pre-eclampsia, but most are incomplete when compared to the full spectrum of the human disease. It also remains to be properly investigated as to whether pre-eclampsia is one disease or a similar manifestation of many disease conditions. This intrigue is fuelled by the two different types of pre-eclampsia: that before 34 weeks and that at or after 34 weeks. Both of these types are completely different: the former has a stormy course that can potentially kill the foetus and mother, whereas the second one seems to be less devastating. Also, their origins seem to be different. Although the former has a placental origin, the latter is genetic in origin. There was a brief period when it was thought that both had nearly same aetiology, and therefore, there was no need to group them separately. However, thankfully, this thinking did not last long. The former is accepted as an obstetric vasculopathy, whereas the latter is not. This brings us to the concept of obstetric vasculopathies.

WHAT IS OBSTETRIC VASCULOPATHY?

In simplest terms, obstetric vasculopathy means a disease of vessels resulting from an obstetric event. Though this is the first step to the understanding of obstetric vasculopathies, it is the most preliminary step. From here, the complexity of this science

begins, and it is this complexity that makes it beautiful but challenging, intriguing and inviting for keen students to decode its mysteries.

Obstetric vasculopathy is not to be confused with vasculitis that occurs in the maternal vascular system. It is the vasculopathy that occurs at the foetomaternal interface. It is, therefore, also known as "placental vasculopathy". Inherited probably by an amorphous genetic propensity at the foetomaternal system, there occurs a series of changes at this interface that invites seemingly totally diverse and apparently unrelated conditions.

In early understandings, it was perceived that one condition led to the other. But as advances in understanding were made, it became clear that these were not cause-and-effect relationships but rather were fruits of the same pathology. In the initial years, only a few conditions were attributed to obstetric vasculopathy, namely:

- Recurrent spontaneous miscarriages (RSA),
- Intrauterine growth restriction (IUGR),
- Pre-eclampsia and pre-eclampsia remote from term,
- Accidental haemorrhage and
- Chorea gravidarum.

However, with scientific research of these conditions, more specifics and complexities added up. Currently, obstetric vasculopathies include:

- RSAs of late first trimesters and second trimesters;
- Accidental haemorrhage with an association of IUGR or pre-eclampsia remote from term and
- Foetal demise of non-anomalous pregnancies with association of any one of the preceding conditions.

Additions to this list also continued to be made and include hyperhomocysteinemia. Systemic lupus erythematosus (SLE)-associated pregnancies are a special class because they have a magnified manifestation of vasculopathy, thereby enabling a closer look at this miraculous but mysterious phenomenon. I am reminded of a thought-provoking incident that took place in 1980. It was during my internship in internal medicine that I witnessed a postgraduate clinical case presentation. A guest faculty visiting the institution was also present during the case presentation of SLE.

This subject was not pregnant and the professor in internal medicine remarked that this was a rare case. The visiting faculty did not agree. He said that he wanted to visit the clinical wards. Much to our surprise, he pointed out many admissions that could have lupus in association (or as I understand it now, an immunological basis). I do not know if any further investigations were done or if it was merely pointed out. But I, too, had completely forgotten this incident until nearly a decade later when I suddenly recollected the event because more and more diverse obstetric conditions started being associated with obstetric vasculopathy. Lest I misunderstood, I wish to clarify that all obstetric vasculopathies are not SLE, but SLE does produce obstetric vasculopathy. I would, however, like to highlight that immunology and its disturbances have a big role to play in obstetric vasculopathy.

PART 2

Possibilities in aetiology of pre-eclampsia

Immunology of pre-eclampsia

IMMUNE TOLERANCE AND PRE-ECLAMPSIA

Obstetric vasculopathies in general and pre-eclampsia, in particular have a strong immunological basis. The foetus is an allograft with half of its immunological component derived from its mother and the other half from the father. The maternal component is her innate, so the mother tolerates it, but the component coming from the father is immunologically distinct, and the maternal system will try to reject it. The conceptus, therefore, needs perpetual protection from the rejection system of the mother. This protection is provided by the paternal immunological component, which seems paradoxical. If the father is immunologically similar to the mother, then his donated organs will be tolerated by the mother, but his foetus will be rejected by her. On the other hand, if he is immunologically different from the mother, his foetus will be well tolerated by the mother, but the organs donated by him will be rejected by the mother. Besides many other protective systems in the mother for the conceptus, syncytiotrophoblasts play an important role as protectors of the conceptus.

In pregnancies where the immune tolerance is suboptimal, a series of effects take place. The premier effect is a defective trophoblastic invasion and this results in clinical conditions known as obstetric vasculopathies. An excessive maternal inflammatory response, directed against foreign foetal antigens results in a chain of events, including shallow trophoblast invasion, defective spiral artery remodelling, placental infarction and release of pro-inflammatory cytokines and placental fragments in the systemic circulation. During a normal pregnancy, trophoblasts interact in the decidua with the unique uterine natural killer (NK) cells, modifying their cytokine repertoire and regulating adhesion molecules and matrix metalloproteinases. The inability of trophoblasts to accomplish these changes might be a critical factor for the onset of pre-eclampsia.[1]

Complete failure of this mechanism can cause miscarriage, and partial failure can cause poor placentation, dysfunctional uteroplacental perfusion and resultant clinical manifestation of obstetric vasculopathies like pre-eclampsia, intrauterine growth restriction (IUGR), and accidental haemorrhage.

TYPES OF PRE-ECLAMPSIA BASED ON IMMUNOLOGY

Pre-eclampsia appears to be two types of diseases:

1. *Pre-eclampsia of onset after 34 weeks*: This type of pre-eclampsia is often indistinguishable from normotensive controls as regards foetomaternal outcomes. In this type of pre-eclampsia, placental malperfusion appears to be minimal. Maternal protective systems that sense the foetus as foreign are kept at bay in normotensive pregnancies that do not register any rise in blood pressure during pregnancy. It does not, however, mean that the maternal systems were not out to eliminate the foetus. But the protective systems successfully thwart its onslaught by the protecting and nourishing mechanisms. It is postulated that

if human pregnancies continue at or beyond 55 weeks, all of them will eventually develop pre-eclampsia. This type of pre-eclampsia has a distinct but amorphous genetic predisposition.

2. *Early onset pre-eclampsia (or pre-eclampsia remote from term)*: This type of pre-eclampsia manifests clinically at or before 34 weeks of pregnancy. It is, therefore, labelled as early-onset pre-eclampsia or pre-eclampsia remote from term. It is acknowledged to be primarily a placental problem, with extensive gross and molecular pathologies causing the release of pro-inflammatory and anti-angiogenic factors into maternal circulation.[2] This type of pre-eclampsia can be stormy and life-threatening for both the mother and the foetus. It is known to be associated with morbidities such as placental abruption, renal failure and can readily progress to eclampsia. This type of pre-eclampsia remains the main focus of all studies, especially for prediction and prevention.

FIRST FEW DAYS OF PLACENTATION AND PRE-ECLAMPSIA

Human pregnancy is often called a two-stage pregnancy. By two stage, it is meant that it is initially maintained by non-placental sources, and by 12 to 14 weeks, the placenta takes over. This does not mean that the placentation process does not begin until 12–14 weeks of human pregnancy because this process is ongoing and robust. It lays the foundation for a healthy obstetric outcome. Events taking place early in pregnancy can have effects as late as at term or just before that. Placental development in the human starts at the time of implantation at or around day 7 post-conception. By day 11 post-conception, the conceptus is already implanted within the shallow or superficial layers of endometrium. By the end of the subsequent week, placental villi cover the total surface of the gestational sac. The placental villi exhibit a bilayer epithelium consisting of cytotrophoblasts with overlaying syncytium (syncytiotrophoblasts). The trophoblasts with well-defined cell walls are called "cytotrophoblasts". Soon, they merge at the tips, leading to the dissolution of the cell walls. These are called "syncytiotrophoblasts". The shell of trophoblasts with syncytiotrophoblasts

at the tip is robust, vital, and alive. It decides the fate of pregnancy in a big way. Events that are to happen after days, weeks or months in an ongoing pregnancy originate here.

The shell with syncytiotrophoblasts at its tip remodels the spiral arterioles of the endometrium. This remodelling is a critical happening. It converts the spiral arterioles into the decidual arterioles. In the bargain, it shields off the vasculature from changes in the maternal systems, thus making the foetoplacental unit autonomous, tightly controlled and self-regulatory.

THE AUTONOMOUS TIGHT UNIT

At this stage early in pregnancy, the autonomous foetomaternal unit does not need any nutrition from the mother nor does it need any extra protection from her. It is so brilliantly devised that it has to essentially function in a hypoxic environment, thereby not needing even oxygen from its mother for survival.

As currently known to science, this tightness and autonomous ambience are necessary because the all-important organogenesis is happening. At the same time, the foetus, a foreign protein for the mother (and therefore, amenable to rejection), is getting tolerated. The maternal system is learning to tolerate the conceptus. With such a critical phenomenon occurring, the foetal unit is kept tightly secured and protected. The mother has hardly any control or influence on this phase.

UTERINE GLANDS AND PLACENTATION

Right from graduate days, students of the subject are taught about the structure and histopathology of the endometrium. Although most teachers detail this efficiently, when it comes to explaining the function of different structures in the uterine endometrium, they tend not do as well. This is because science itself has not revealed the details of the functions of the structures that constitute the endometrium. Good quality research in recent years has revealed some mysteries of uterine glands and their functions.

It has now been shown that the endometrial glands have a critical function of synthesising, transporting and secreting the nutrition essential for the early conceptus in nearly all mammals.

Studies on human conceptus have ethical constraints, and as a result, many of the conclusions are drawn from other mammalian species like mice and ewes.

Filant and Spencer describe the morphogenetic events common to the post-conception events in the uterus.[3] These events include:

1. Organisation and stratification of the endometrial stroma,
2. Differentiation and growth of myometrium and
3. Coordinated development of uterine glands.

The evidence that uterine glands and their secretions are critical for supporting early pregnancy has been discovered as recently as in last decade.[4]

Uterine milk

In 1959, it was Needham who formally coined the term "uterine milk" for the secretions of uterine glands. It was because of the nourishment that these secretions provide to the early conceptus.[5] The human placenta is haemochorial placenta, meaning it is a type of placenta in which the maternal blood is in direct contact with the chorion. Though haemochorial, in human placenta (vis-à-vis other mammals) foetal villi do not float uncovered in the maternal blood. They are surrounded by endometrial (decidual) cells that secrete a fluid, which nourishes the conceptus and is, therefore, called "uterine milk". This was stated as early as in 1884 by Von Hoffman.[6] It now appears that the influence of uterine milk is not only confined to the nutrition of the conceptus but also for healthy implantation. Understandably, therefore, problems in this process can cause recurrent pregnancy loss and infertility.

Having introduced the term "uterine milk", one more term needs an introduction – histotrophs. The term "histotroph" means "the total of all nutrient material derived from maternal tissues other than from maternal blood and is used by the embryo for its survival and nourishment". Histotrophy originally indicated the additional nourishment that the embryo receives beyond that from the maternal blood, but scientific research has proven that early in human pregnancy, it is not the additional nutrition but the only and critical nutrition that the conceptus receives. The hematogenous source of maternal nutrition becomes accessible only at and after 12–14 weeks.

Uterine milk also contains carbohydrates, lipids, and amino acids, which together provide a rich source of the energy needed to support the rapid proliferation of cells. Uterine milk also contains a variety of growth factors that stimulate the proliferation and growth activity of the trophoblasts.

Uterine gland knockout cells

Uterine gland knockout (UGKO) epithelial cells has proven to be useful in the understanding of the foetoplacental unit in early pregnancy. Understanding UGKO has come from experiments in pregnant ewes. It has been found that the epithelial cells and their secretory activities can be efficiently blocked by progestins. The hypothesis that progestins can block the uterine glandular activity was tested by Bartol et al. in 1988.[7] They exposed ewes to norgestimate, a potent synthetic progestin, from their birth to postnatal day 13 and found that the uterine adenogenesis was successfully inhibited. Exposure of the neonatal ewes to norgestimate did not hamper the gross development of Müllerian system. Additionally, norgestimate did not affect the development of the brain or the hypothalamo-pituitary-ovarian axis, but it decisively blocked the development of the glandular component in the endometrium. This resulted in infertility or subsequent miscarriages in the ewes. Results from these studies explained the critical role of uterine glands in the secretion of uterine milk and a subsequent healthy pregnancy outcome.

The uterine glands express genes that encode for secretory factors, amino acid transporters, glucose transporters, migration and attachment factors, regulators of calcium, phosphorus homeostasis, secreted peptidase, protease inhibitors, and immune-modulatory factor. The process of gene encoding evolved and alters the intrauterine environment, making it conducive to successful implantation and subsequent growth of the conceptus.[8-11] The profound changes that take place in the endometrial gland during pregnancy also allow for the increase in secretory requirements of its glands. These secretions are transported to the foetus through specialised areas in the placenta of the studied mammals. They are known as "areola".[12]

Most of the contents of uterine milk are nutritive amino acids, which also have other developmental functions. Uterine milk includes stepwise development of the early embryo as well as the migration of primitive structures to right positions like the trophectoderm. Any disturbance in this can disrupt the milieu, resulting in early pregnancy loss. It is also possible that adverse functioning of these pregnancy-supporting structures can also produce its effects on the activity of the trophoblasts and can subsequently increase the possibility of pre-eclampsia. Thus, deficient glandular activity is hypothesised to be responsible for early pregnancy loss or other subsequent complications.

Many of these mechanisms have their basis in animal experiments, and one would to know if such a mechanism operates in humans as well. Circumstantial evidence strongly indicates it to be a possibility, and this is particularly true for the interesting phenomenon of blastocyst-decidual crosstalk.

The crosstalk

This entire process of trophoblastic generation, growth and proliferation, which ultimately results in the generation of a healthy placenta needs dialogue for crosstalk between the blastocyst and the decidua. Burton and Jauniaux rightly called it "a fascinating paradigm".[2] It is well-established now that the maternal immune system and the placenta are involved in the highly choreographed crosstalk that causes adequate spiral artery remodelling, which is required for uteroplacental perfusion and the free flow of nutrients to the foetus.[13]

The maternal circulation in and through the placental bed is established towards the end of the first trimester (about 11–13 weeks of pregnancy). Until then, the nutrition of the conceptus is maintained through endometrial glands. These secretions are produced, transported and delivered into the cavity of the placenta. The early and young villi are bathed in these secretions, and so are the trophoblasts.

One question that can arise at this stage is: What maintains the supply of the trophoblasts? The answer to this is also interesting. Trophoblasts send signals to the endometrial glands and upregulate growth factors. This is a function of the blastocyst-endometrial crosstalk. These growth factors include epidermal growth factor (EGF),

fibroblast growth factor-2 (FGF2) and insulin-like growth factor-1 (IGF1). In bovine experimental studies, cooperative interactions for EGF, FGF and IGF1 on the proliferation of the bovine trophoblast cell line and resultant bovine embryo development has been clearly shown.[14] All these factors are in turn required for trophoblast stem cells, which are the source for the supply of trophoblasts.

This concept of crosstalk came originally from animal experiments. The endometrial gland cells display the same array of endocrine receptors as are expressed in animal species, and pathologists have long recognised the hypersecretory phenotype that the glands adopt early in pregnancy, the so-called Arias-Stella reaction. Lower levels of glycoproteins secreted by the glands, such as glycodelin-A, have been linked to miscarriage because in 70% of cases, formation of the trophoblastic shell is incomplete.[2] Furthermore, microarray analysis of chorionic villus samples from patients that went on to develop pre-eclampsia show aberrant expression of decidual, rather than placental, genes.[15] It is indeed possible that the defective dialogue leads to defective placentation and, subsequently, to the development of pre-eclampsia.

Currently, measures in the prevention of pre-eclampsia are confined to the prevention of effects. It is possible that if this system is exactly decoded and the algorithm operating in the placentation correctly identified, prevention of the cause of pre-eclampsia can become a distinct possibility in the future.

REFERENCES

1. Matthiesen L, Berg G, Ernerudh J, Ekerfelt C, Jonsson Y, Sharma S: Immunology of preeclampsia. *Chem Immunol Allergy* 89:49–61, 2005.
2. Burton GJ, Jauniaux E: The cytotrophoblastic shell and complications of pregnancy. *Placenta* 60:134–139, 2017.
3. Filant J, Spencer TE: Uterine glands: Biological roles in conceptus implantation, uterine receptivity, and decidualization. *Int J Dev Biol* 58:107–116, 2014. doi:10.1387/ijdb.130344ts.
4. Cooke PS, Ekman GC, Kaur J, Davila J, Bagchi IC, Clark SG, Dziuk PJ, Hayashi K, Bartol FF: Brief exposure to progesterone

during a critical neonatal window prevents uterine gland formation in mice. *Biol Reprod* 86:63, 2012.

5. Needham J. *A History of Embryology*, 1959, London, UK, Cambridge University Press.

6. Von Hoffman G: Uterine milk. *Am J Med Sci* 87:254–255, 1884.

7. Bartol FF, Wiley AA, Coleman DA, Wolfe DF, Riddell MG: Ovine uterine morphogenesis: Effects of age and progestin administration and withdrawal on neonatal endometrial development and DNA synthesis. *J Anim Sci* 66:3000–3009, 1988.

8. Bazer FW, Wu G, Spencer TE, Johnson GA, Burghardt RC, Bayless K: Novel pathways for implantation and establishment and maintenance of pregnancy in mammals. *Mol Hum Reprod* 16:135–152, 2010.

9. Dorniak P, Bazer FW, Spencer TE: Physiology and Endocrinology Symposium: Biological role of interferon tau in endometrial function and conceptus elongation. *J Anim Sci* 91:1627–1638, 2013.

10. Forde N, Lonergan P: Transcriptomic analysis of the bovine endometrium: What is required to establish uterine receptivity to implantation in cattle? *J Reprod Dev* 58:189–195, 2012.

11. Spencer TE, Sandra O, Wolf E: Genes involved in conceptus-endometrial interactions in ruminants: Insights from reductionism and thoughts on holistic approaches. *Reproduction* 135:165–179, 2008.

12. Burton GJ, Scioscia M, Rademacher TW: Endometrial secretions: Creating a stimulatory microenvironment within the human early placenta and implications for the aetiopathogenesis of preeclampsia. *J Reprod Immunol* 89:118–125, 2011.

13. Peixoto AB, Rolo LC, Nardozza LMM, Araujo Júnior E: Epigenetics and preeclampsia: Programming of future outcomes. *Methods Mol Biol* 1710:73–83, 2018. doi:10.1007/978-1-4939-7498-6_6.

14. Xie M, McCoski SR, Johnson SE, Rhoads ML, Ealy AD: Combinatorial effects of epidermal growth factor, fibroblast growth factor 2 and insulin-like growth factor 1 on trophoblast cell proliferation and embryogenesis in cattle. *Reprod Fertil Dev* 29(2):419–430, 2017. doi:10.1071/RD15226.

15. Conrad KP, Rabaglino MB, Post Uiterweer ED: Emerging role for dysregulated decidualization in the genesis of preeclampsia. *Placenta* 60:119–129, 2017.

3

Endothelial cell dysfunction and pre-eclampsia

INTRODUCTION

One constant feature mentioned in the aetiopathology of pre-eclampsia is endothelial cell dysfunction. Endothelial cells line the entire vascular bed (Figure 3.1) and are located between the vascular smooth muscles in the vessel wall and the flowing blood column (Figure 3.2). The endothelial cells form a one-cell layer wall called the "endothelium". It lines all blood vessels, including the arteries, arterioles, venules, veins and capillaries. The capillaries, however, are entirely lined by the endothelium (Figure 3.3). There is no smooth muscle lining below the endothelium in the capillaries.

All secretions and releases from these cells consequently have direct access to the entire body through blood. In turn, they also have a vulnerability. Because of this strategic location and resultant access to diverse circulating substances, endothelial cells can directly modulate the tone of the vessels. Along with this, they also modulate the processes of coagulation and vascular permeability. Vascular tone is maintained by endothelial cells striking a balance between the circulating vasodilatory and vasoconstrictive substances. The body needs a potent, well-balanced and well-toned vascular system. It achieves this by modulating the tone of the vessel musculature. As has been previously mentioned, the blood does not come in direct contact with vessel walls and, therefore, is relatively remote from the smooth muscles lining them. Endothelial cells are interceding between the vessel walls and the circulating blood column.

In pre-eclampsia, the vascular tone plays an important role. It is maintained by striking a balance between vasoconstrictive and vasodilatory substances. The most well-known vasoconstrictive substances active in pregnancy are endothelin and TXA_2, and the most potent vasodilatory substances are NO and PGI_2.

In the same way as maintaining a balance between dilatory and constrictive substances leads to maintaining vascular tone, the flow of blood without coagulating is maintained by procoagulants and anticoagulants in circulation. The vascular permeability is controlled by endothelial cells maintaining the tightness of endothelial cell junctions. Excessively weak cell junctions lead to tissue oedema as the permeability of vessel wall increases as is seen in pre-eclampsia.

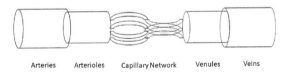

Arteries   Arterioles   Capillary Network   Venules   Veins

Figure 3.1 Vascular bed.

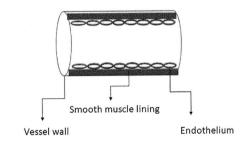

Smooth muscle lining

Vessel wall   Endothelium

Figure 3.2 Schematic representation of arteries, arterioles, veins and venules.

15

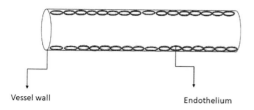

Figure 3.3 Schematic representation of capillary wall.

THE PHENOMENON OF ENDOTHELIAL CELL ACTIVATION

Endothelial cell activation is a unique phenomenon. It occurs in the endothelial cells when they are subjected to sublethal injury. This activation process is characteristically found in the generation of atherosclerosis in the body. The phenomenon of endothelial cell activation in the non-pregnant state is different from that of one in pregnancy. Pregnancy-related endothelial cell activation is typically characterised by higher levels of both coagulation endothelial markers and endothelial activation markers like Matrix Matalloproteinases (MMPs). In pregnancy, changes in extracellular matrix composition and MMP activity also occur and promote vascular remodelling in the uterus.[1]

Endothelial cell activation provoked many to suggest that pre-eclampsia in particular and obstetric vasculopathies in general are a result of inflammation and transient atherosclerotic process. Nevertheless, the two have been found to have a small but significant contributory role in the entire complex plethora of aetiopathology of pre-eclampsia. Endothelial cell dysfunction and resultant activation in pre-eclampsia results from a variety of factors. These include physical shearing forces, hypoxia or ROS and their metabolites and other circulating constituents.[2]

Flow conditions critically regulate endothelial cell functions in the vasculature. Reduced shear stress resulting from disturbed blood flow can drive the development of vascular inflammatory lesions.[3] Vasospasm generated in pre-eclampsia can cause the tearing or shearing force on the endothelial cells, leading to their activation. Vasospasm generates a hypoxic microenvironment explaining its contribution to endothelial cell activation. ROS, as well as its denatured products, are abundant in circulation

in pre-eclampsia. These denatured products include peroxidised LDL and peroxidised VLDL moieties of lipids. All three together in synchrony – the shearing force, hypoxia and circulating oxidised products lead to endothelial cell activation.

The process of endothelial cell activation may occur at the foetomaternal interface or can occur in the entire maternal vasculature. This could be seen in two clinical entities of obstetric vasculopathies: Pre-eclampsia and intrauterine growth restriction (IUGR). In pre-eclampsia, the activation of endothelial cells occurs throughout the body systems, and in IUGR, it is confined to the foetomaternal interface.

Renal glomerular capillary endotheliosis is one entity where endothelial cell activation takes place in pre-eclampsia in the renal system. It represents a specific variant of thrombotic microangiopathy. It is characterised by glomerular endothelial swelling with a loss of endothelial fenestrae and the occlusion of the capillary lumens. Unusually, thrombosis may also be found. Recent evidence suggests that this glomerular lesion is mediated by a soluble VEGF receptor that deprives glomerular endothelial cells of the VEGF. This leads to cellular injury and disruption of the filtration apparatus with subsequent proteinuria.[4] Similar lesions attributable to endothelial cell activation have been described in other organs of the body of a person who is pre-eclamptic. This includes lesions in the liver, uterus and extra-uterine organ systems and tissues.

CIRCULATING MARKERS OF ENDOTHELIAL ACTIVATION

Many markers have been identified in experimental and clinical investigations, which are supposed to indicate the endothelial activation process. They have been reported in pre-eclampsia and include:

- Increased circulating concentration of endothelin-1.[5]
- Increased levels of fibronectin in circulation.[6]
- Decreased levels of circulating vasodilator PGI_2.[7]
- Altered levels of circulating thrombomodulin.[8]

ENDOTHELIAL ACTIVATION AND PROSTAGLANDINS

Prostaglandins are acknowledged as important markers of endothelial cell activation. During normal pregnancy, there is an important balance between vasoconstrictive prostaglandins like TXA$_2$ with vasodilatory prostaglandins like PGI$_2$. Throughout pregnancy, the bias of the female body is towards PGI$_2$. But in pre-eclampsia, PGI$_2$ levels reduce and TXA$_2$ levels increase. This is reflected in the plasma urinary secretion of PGI$_2$ getting reduced in pre-eclampsia.[7]

Altered prostaglandin production results from the circulating peroxidised lipid molecules in pre-eclampsia. Denatured lipids directly affect the cyclooxygenase pathway that is so critical in generating prostaglandins from arachidonic acid. Placentas from subjects with pre-eclampsia are known to produce more TXA$_2$ and peroxidised lipids when compared with normal placenta. It seems that endothelial cell activation is one of the resultant insults of this aetiopathology.

The process of endothelial cell activation is not the only change contributing to the aetiopathology of pre-eclampsia. The cellular and chemical manifestation of this process provide many useful markers in the prediction of pre-eclampsia and its allied adverse obstetric outcomes. It seems that endothelial cell activation following a series of sublethal injuries provide the ROS needed for the process of lipid peroxidation that is taking place in the intercellular matrix.

If this entire aetiopathology is to be summarised at this stage, it could be done thus: Functional slowing of maternal blood pool at the foetomaternal interface leads to shearing force at the level of endothelium. This results in endothelial cell activation. The VLDL and dense small lipid particles of LDL tend to walk in and out of the intercellular matrix. Consequent to the process of endothelial cell activation, when the lipids walk into the intercellular matrix, they come in close contact with the ROS released by the activated endothelial cells. These ROS then peroxidise or in simpler terms, denature the lipid particles. The lipid particles that are so denatured when going back to the circulation serve as agents of free radicals. Wherever the denatured lipids go, they activate the endothelial cells and, at the same time, initiate the cyclooxygenase pathway alterations in such a way that TXA$_2$ release is increased. This leads to vasospasm and consequent clinical manifestations of pre-eclampsia.

PLASMINOGEN AND ALLIED PROCOAGULANT ACTIVITY: A MANIFESTATION OF ENDOTHELIAL CELL ACTIVATION

Any cell is a complete structure with a series of life-sustaining and life-protecting mechanisms in place for its survival. Sublethal injuries that lead to endothelial cell activation produce a plethora of changes and releases. One of these is a release of plasminogen proteins and plasminogen activation. It is well-known from basic human physiology that plasminogen is one of the final critical steps that subsequently leads to the formation of plasmin, which is necessary for the ultimate formation of a coagulum or a thrombus.

Endothelial cell activation leads to an increase in PAI-1. In pregnancies uncomplicated by pre-eclampsia, PAI-1 is reduced at the foetomaternal interface, which leads to reduced thrombosis and good quality of blood circulation at the foetomaternal interface. Increase in PAI-1 has been well-documented in pre-eclampsia.[9] Circulating levels of PAI-1 were found to be directly correlated with the severity of pre-eclampsia.[10] Such a close association between PAI-1 and pre-eclampsia led to studying its role in predicting pre-eclampsia. It was found that when combined with uterine artery Doppler, it can help predict pre-eclampsia.[11]

ANTIPHOSPHOLIPID ANTIBODIES ACT THROUGH PROCOAGULANT MECHANISM

In a wide spectrum of immunological causes of obstetric vasculopathies, antiphospholipid antibodies are known to be a leading cause. They are believed to be acting through a procoagulant action. Other procoagulant molecules have also been subsequently identified to be acting similar to antiphospholipid antibodies in pregnancy. In a series of obstetric vasculopathy leading to pre-eclampsia remote from term, 25% of women had functional protein S deficiency, 18% demonstrated hyperhomocysteinemia and 29% had detectable levels of antiphospholipid antibodies in one study.[12] These molecules appear to get functionally affected, leading to endothelial cell activation. These in turn produce an imbalance of pro- and anticoagulation milieu in a pregnant woman in favour of procoagulants. As a result, there is an activation of the entire cycle of the aetiopathology of obstetric vasculopathies. The molecules like antiphospholipid antibodies can activate the endothelial cells at the foetomaternal interface early in a pregnancy, leading to foetal demise and subsequent miscarriage.

ENDOTHELIAL CELL ADHESION MOLECULE DISTURBANCES

The process of endothelial cell activation following sublethal injury leads to a series of changes at the foetomaternal interface as well as in the entire maternal vasculature. The procoagulation-anticoagulation balance being disturbed in favour of procoagulation has been examined in the preceding section. One more change that occurs as a result of endothelial cell activation is the release or activation of some specific cell adhesion molecules. Two principle cell molecules that have been identified are fibronectin and von Willebrand Factor (VWF).

The ultrastructure of fibronectin gives a valuable insight resulting from endothelial cell activation. Studies have clearly shown that a rise in fibronectin levels precedes clinical manifestation of pre-eclampsia, and an endothelial vascular injury is a primary event in the genesis of pre-eclampsia.[13] The fibronectin molecules remain in the extracellular matrix close to the endothelial cells. Their ultrastructure study reveals that they have a fibrillary structure. During the process of endothelial cell activation, this fibrillary structure gets disturbed or distorted. Because of this distortion, there is a loss of a chymotryptic protease-sensitive isotope. This in turn precipitates a further loss of fibronectin fibrillary structure, thereby generating a vicious cycle. The loss of fibronectin fibrillary structure leads to the activation of neutrophils, which in turn leads to amplified destruction of fibronectin fibrillary structure. The vicious circle thus gets amplified and perpetuated. Endothelial cell activation, besides leading to fibronectin ultrastructure disturbance, also leads to the proactive secretion of fibronectin and molecules like VWF from the activated endothelial cells. It seems that hypoxia also has an important role in this process.

The process of active secretion of these molecules provides the supply chain of fibronectin to the fire of endothelial cell activation by interleukin-1. The constant supply of fibronectin that is required to sustain this vicious cycle is provided by the activated endothelial cells. This is how the process is activated, perpetuated and amplified. Besides these pathophysiological consequences, alteration in fibronectin levels serves as a useful marker for endothelial injury. Elevated fibronectin means an active vicious circle, which means there are endothelial injury and resultant cell activation.[14]

VEGF

Pre-eclampsia, as is well-known, has major alteration in the angiogenic process. This involves an inadequate vascular dilation and remodelling of spiral arteries. The VEGF is necessary for modulating the angiogenic processes in the placenta. The reduction of VEGF in pre-eclampsia leads to hypoperfusion and subsequent hypoxia of the foetus in hypertensive pregnancy VEGF alterations increase vascular permeability. In some cases, VEGF is also called "vascular permeability factor" because it plays an important role in increasing vascular permeability in pre-eclampsia. Considerably high levels of VEGF have indeed been demonstrated.[15]

Further detailing this increase in VEGF was done to identify the source, and it was found that VEGF in pre-eclampsia is not of placental origin but of maternal vascular origin. The VEGF levels rapidly increased when retinal epithelial cells were exposed to molecules of oxidative stress like superoxide or hydrogen peroxides.[16] But another study showed that there are placental regional changes and the central foetal region of the placenta contributes an increase in VEGF.[17] These two conflicting studies create controversy as to whether VEGF is of a maternal or foetal source. However, hypoxic conditions in the placenta precipitating an increase in VEGF levels seem to be agreed upon.

Clinical bearings

Obstetric vasculopathies like IUGR and abruptio placenta wherein the aetiopathology is confined to the placenta, there is no clinical oedema found. Although in pre-eclampsia, where the process involves the entire maternal vasculature, oedema is seen in clinical practice. VEGF seems to be released by the activated endothelial cells of maternal vasculature. Therefore in conditions where endothelial cells of maternal vasculature are not involved, there is no increase in vascular permeability, and as a result, there is no oedema.

It is of interest that circulating levels of VEGF are not increased by worsening pre-eclampsia. Also, no correlation has been found between the levels of VEGF and obstetric outcome in pre-eclampsia. Therefore, VEGF is not a good prognosticator in pre-eclampsia.

ENDOTHELIN

One more circulating protein in pre-eclampsia associated with the process of endothelial activation is endothelin. Endothelin is a 21-amino acid peptide that is produced by the vascular endothelium from a 39-amino acid precursor, through the actions of an endothelin converting enzyme (ECE) found on the endothelial cell membrane. Endothelin has different subtypes. The subtype Endothelin-1 (ET-1) is the most potent vasoconstrictor in the pregnant woman. ET-1, like all forms of endothelin, is released by the activated endothelial cells. But ET-1 is not found in circulation before pre-eclampsia becomes clinically evident. Therefore, it has no predictive value. However, it is believed to have a key role as a mediator of hypertension in pre-eclampsia.[18]

Also, ET-1 is not found to have a placental origin. This characteristic of ET-1 is similar to VEGF. ET-1 levels were studied in blood from a uterine vein and an antecubital vein. The former is blood from the placental origin and the latter from the general vascular bed. It was found that ET-1 levels were distinctly higher in the antecubital blood. However, they were negligible in the blood collected from the uterine vein.[19] This proves that the source of ET-1 is non-placental. Maternal endothelial cells, when sublethally injured and activated, release ET-1. Placenta has no role to play in this. It is possible that TXA_2 that is released because of endothelial activation and resultant lipid peroxidation initiates the vasospasm in pre-eclampsia. Therefore, the vasospasm generated at the foeto-maternal interface is attributable to TXA_2/PGI_2

balance getting tipped in favour of TXA_2. However, for subsequent maintenance and even amplification of the process of vasospasm, ET-1 steps in. It generates vasospasm in the entire maternal vessel bed and produces its clinical complications and manifestations of pre-eclampsia.

OTHER MOLECULES CONTRIBUTING TO ENDOTHELIAL CELL ACTIVATION

The endothelial cell activation process can be compared to an orchestra because it is not a chain of events, but the activators act in quick rhythmic succession that results in endothelial cell activation. Although many such molecules have been identified, it is possible that these are not the only ones. There may be still some unknown molecules, which also may contribute to the process of decidual cell activation. The biggest players in this game, however, are the oxidised lipid molecules – LDL and VLDL.

The others are described as immunological antibodies, cytokines, formed elements in blood and toxins.

Immunological antibodies

Amongst these immunologically active molecules, the antiphospholipid antibodies cause direct endothelial cell activation. Elevated levels of Immunoglobulin G (IgG) and Immunoglobulin M (IgM) antibodies have been consistently reported in women with pre-eclampsia remote from term. It is worthwhile noting that a separate evaluation of IgG and IgM antibodies does not have any clinical significance especially with regard to antiphospholipid antibodies. The two only indicate the avidity of these antibodies because their clinical effects are similar.

Cytokines

Cytokines have long had the attention of investigators in pre-eclampsia. A series of such "destructive" cytokines have been identified, which also cause endothelial cell activation. The principal player in this family is Tumor Necrosis Factor Alpha (TNF-α).

Formed elements in blood

A series of cellular components of blood have also been found to play an important role in the process of decidual cell activation. These include:

- Platelets,
- Neutrophils, and
- Placenta Membrane Microvesicles.

"Toxins"

Historically, pre-eclampsia was called "pre-eclamptic toxaemia": or even plain and simple "toxaemia". This was because the assumption that by some mechanism, toxins are released by the placenta, which led to the development of pre-eclampsia. It was subsequently disproved because no such toxin was identified in the circulation of pre-eclamptic women. This led to a change in name from pre-eclamptic toxaemia to pre-eclampsia. Nevertheless, inspired by those early presumptions, some researchers indulge in attempting to identify or, at least, search for the ever-elusive toxin, even now. Such efforts have also been made in the possible agents ("toxins") that might cause decidual or maternal vascular endothelial cell activation.

Metallothionein has been proposed as a toxic factor that may cause endothelial cell activation. However, there are more questions than answers to metallothionein and its action on the endothelium. It is believed that metallothionein binds with circulating cadmium to produce a complex cadmium-metallothionein. Manifestations of cadmium toxicity lead to a syndrome similar to pre-eclampsia.[20] Though it was exhibited as the possible toxin that produced "pre-eclamptic toxaemia", it did not find much support in the scientific world.

However, there is no denying that endothelial cell activation plays a major role in pre-eclampsia, but pre-eclampsia is caused and influenced by many factors. Understanding the complexity of factors and intricacies of endothelial activation can hold the key to treating pre-eclampsia.

LIST OF ABBREVIATIONS

ET-1	endothelin-1
IgG	immunoglobulin G
LDL	low density lipoprotein
MMPs	matrix metalloproteinases
NO	nitric oxide
PAI-1	plasminogen activator inhibitor-1
PGI_2	prostaglandin I_2
ROS	reactive oxygen species
TNF-α	tumor necrosis factor alpha
TXA_2	thromboxane A_2
VEGF	vascular endothelial growth factor
VLDL	very-low-density lipoprotein
VWF	von Willebrand factor

REFERENCES

1. Slavik L, Prochazkova J, Prochazka M, Simetka O, Hlusi A, Ulehlova J: The pathophysiology of endothelial function in pregnancy and the usefulness of endothelial markers. *Biomed Pap Med Fac Univ Palacky Olomouc Czech Repub* 155(4):333–337, 2011.
2. de Groot C, Taylor R: New insights into the etiology of preeclampsia. *Ann Med* 25(3):243–249, 1993.
3. Babendreyer A, Molls L, Dreymueller D, Uhlig S, Ludwig A: Shear stress counteracts endothelial CX3CL1 induction and monocytic cell adhesion. *Mediators Inflamm* 2017:1515389, 2017. doi:10.1155/2017/1515389. Epub 2017 Mar 26.
4. Stillman IE, Karumanch SA: The glomerular injury of preeclampsia. *J Am Soc Nephrol* 18:2281–2284, 2007. doi:10.1681/ASN.2007020255.
5. Bakrania B, Duncan J, Warrington JP, Granger JP: The endothelin type a receptor as a potential therapeutic target in pre-eclampsia. *Int J Mol Sci* 18(3):E522, 2017. doi:10.3390/ijms18030522.
6. Taylor R, Crombleholme W, Friedman S: High plasma cellular levels correlate with biochemical and clinical features of pre-eclampsia but cannot be attributed to hypertension alone. *Am J Obstet Gynecol* 165:895–901, 1991.
7. Remuzzi G, Marchesi D, Zoja C, Muratore D, Mecca G, Misiani R, Rossi E et al.: Reduced umbilical and placental vascular prostacyclin in severe preeclampsia. *Prostaglandins* 20(1):105–110, 1980.
8. Turner RJ, Bloemenkamp KW, Bruijn JA, Baelde HJ: Loss of thrombomodulin in placental dysfunction in

preeclampsia. *Arterioscler Thromb Vasc Biol* 36(4):728–735, 2016. doi:10.1161/ATVBAHA.115.306780. Epub 2016 Feb 18.

9. Paidas M, Haut M, Lockwood C: Platelet disorders in pregnancy: Implications for mother and fetus. *Mt Sinai J Med* 61(5):389–403, 1994.

10. Shaarawy M, Didy H: Thrombomodulin, plasminogen activator inhibitor type 1 (PAI-1) and fibronectin as biomarkers of endothelial damage in preeclampsia and eclampsia. *Int J Gynecol Obstet* 55(2):135–139, 1996.

11. Bodova KB, Biringer K, Dokus K, Ivankova J, Stasko J, Danko J: Fibronectin, plasminogen activator inhibitor type 1 (PAI-1) and uterine artery Doppler velocimetry as markers of preeclampsia. *Dis Markers* 30(4):191–196, 2011. doi:10.3233/DMA-2011-0772.

12. Dekker G, de Vries J, Doelitzsch P, Huijgens P, von Blomberg B, Jakobs C, van Geijn H: Underlying disorders associated with severe early-onset preeclampsia. *Am J Obstet Gynecol* 173(4):1042–1048, 1995.

13. Lockwood CJ, Peters JH: Increased plasma levels of ED1+ cellular fibronectin precede the clinical signs of preeclampsia. *Am J Obstet Gynecol* 162(2):358–362, 1990.

14. Forsyth K, Levinsky R: Fibronectin degradation; an in-vitro model of neutrophil mediated endothelial cell damage. *J Pathol* 161(4):313–319, 1990.

15. Kurtoglu E, Avci B, Kokcu A, Celik H, Cengiz Dura M, Malatyalioglu E, Zehra Ozdemir A: Serum VEGF and PGF may be significant markers in prediction of severity of pre-eclampsia. *J Matern Fetal Neonatal Med* 29(12):1987–1992, 2016. doi:10.3109/14767058.2015.1072157.

16. Kuroki M, Voest E, Amano S, Beerepoot L, Takashima S, Tolentino M, Kim R et al.: Reactive oxygen intermediates increase vascular endothelial growth factor expression in vitro and in vivo. *J Clin Invest* 98(7):1667–1675, 1996.

17. Sahay AS, Jadhav AT, Sundrani DP, Wagh GN, Mehendale SS, Chavan-Gautam P, Joshi SR: VEGF and VEGFR1 levels in different regions of the normal and preeclampsia placentae. *Mol Cell Biochem* 438(1–2):141–152, 2018. doi:10.1007/s11010-017-3121-y. Epub 2017 Aug 2.

18. George EM, Granger JP: Endothelin: Key mediator of hypertension in preeclampsia. *Am J Hypertens* 24(9):964–969, 2011. doi:10.1038/ajh.2011.99.

19. Rust O, Bofill J, Zappe D, Hall J, Burnett J Jr, Martin J Jr: The origin of endothelin-1 in patients with severe preeclampsia. *Obstet Gynecol* 89(5 Pt 1):754–757, 1997.

20. Chisolm J, Handorf C: Further observations on the etiology of preeclampsia: Mobilization of toxic cadmium-metallothionein into the serum during pregnancy. *Med Hypotheses* 47(2):123–128, 1996.

4

Oxidative stress and pre-eclampsia

INTRODUCTION

Towards the end of last millennium, oxidative stress was considered to be on the fringe of some disease processes. Nevertheless, interest in this process was already kindled, and many research activities around the globe began looking at the complexities of oxidative stress and its role in the causation of some critical diseases. As details emerged from careful research, it appeared that oxidative stress and immunological changes seem to be partners in the crime. When immunology lays the foundation of pre-eclampsia, oxidative stress perpetuates it. However, these friends are not averse to changing roles. During the ongoing process, oxidative stress can become the cause and immunological processes switching over its role to perpetuator of the process of pre-eclampsia.

WHAT IS OXIDATIVE STRESS?

In nature, countless forces have counter-forces that neutralize each other. To understand this, one may look at Chinese philosophy: yin and yang ("negative-positive") describe how seemingly opposite or contrary forces may be complementary, interconnected and interdependent in the natural world. When these forces remain in balance, peace (health) prevails. However, in the absence of one, the other gets unbalanced and can produce a havoc. This model can help us understand the process of oxidative stress.

At this stage, it is wise to introduce the term "free radical". To start, a free radical is like the yin. It needs a yang to balance it. Yang can be compared to reducing systems. In health, the free radicals remain in balance with the reducing systems. If this balance gets disturbed, many diseases can occur and it includes pre-eclampsia.

WHAT IS A FREE RADICAL?

To understand free radicals easily, we will visit the atomic model that was taught to us in schools. Each atom is made of extremely tiny particles called "protons", "neutrons" and "electrons". Protons and neutrons are in the centre of the atom, making up the nucleus. Electrons surround the nucleus (Figure 4.1). Protons have a positive charge. Electrons have a negative charge. The charge on the proton and electron are the same size but opposite. Neutrons have no charge. Because opposite charges attract, protons and electrons attract each other. Many new subatomic particles have since been added. The neutrinos and the bosons are some of them. However, for our understanding, the role of free radicals in health and diseases, the simplest model of electrons, protons and neutrons will suffice.

Free radicals are also known as "reactive oxygen species" (ROS). These are atoms that have an unpaired electron (Figure 4.2). On the other hand, the reducing systems are atoms that have an unpaired proton. A free radical is like an unbalanced powerful force. The reducing systems that have an extra or

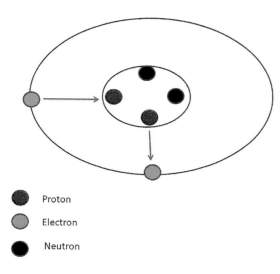

Figure 4.1 A balanced atom.

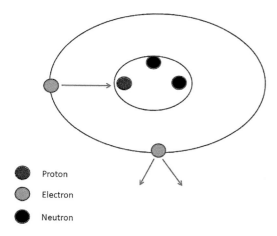

Figure 4.2 A free radical.

un-neutralized proton provide that electron to the free radical, thereby neutralizing it (Figure 4.3). If not effectively and timely neutralized, free radicals can produce extensive changes and a series of pathological manifestations. These are disease processes as a result of oxidative stress.

OXYGEN: A DOUBLE-EDGED SWORD

As children, since the time that we are taught about the goodness, usefulness and life-promoting characteristics of oxygen, we develop a great respect, bordering on veneration for oxygen. It is only when we go for higher studies, we realize that oxygen is not universally kind to everyone and every matter on earth. Even to human beings, it can be devastating. Our white blood cells use oxygen to kill invading bacteria. For those bacteria, oxygen is a killing agent. That oxygen is fundamentally toxic often comes as a surprise to those of us who find it so friendly to our well-being. To other things, it is a terror. It is what turns butter rancid and makes iron rust. Even we as humans can only tolerate it up to a point. The oxygen level in our cells is only about a tenth the level found in the atmosphere. If oxygen levels rise beyond the permissible limits, which it usually does at the cost of carbon dioxide, alarm bells start ringing. This is why anaesthesiologists who administer anaesthesia for endoscopy measures carbon dioxide with monitors; they not only want carbon dioxide in the human body but that at permissible levels, never letting it fall to low levels, because falling levels also means rising oxygen.

One can, therefore, easily philosophise and say that there is nothing universal about goodness or evil of anyone or anything. Some things are good to some and evil to others. Also, good things are good in one situation and can be evil at others or to the same beings in a different situation. In an anaerobic (or non-oxygen-using) world, oxygen is extremely poisonous. Anaerobic organisms abhor oxygen. There is nothing more lethal to them than oxygen. No wonder they have retreated deep inside the dark depths of our intestines where oxygen cannot reach them, letting them survive – and what a survival it is. These organisms are our friends. They help digest our food deep inside our gut.

An oxygen atom can generate a devastating process called "oxidative stress". Its habit of rendering butter rancid in the kitchen continues inside the body. Lipids seem to be a delicacy relished by oxygen. In the body vasculature, the excited form of oxygen known as ROS feasts on the lipids and can cause profound effects in the human system. We shall this in detail in the pages that follow.

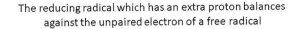

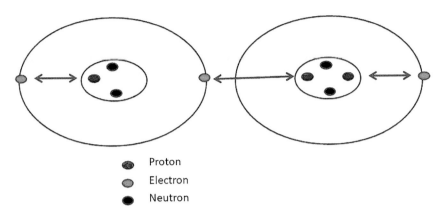

Figure 4.3 Reducing systems mechanism.

THE MISCHIEF OF FREE RADICALS IN VASCULAR WALLS

Pregnancy reminds one of a wrestling ring. The fight begins from day one and goes on until the pregnancy is over. The fight is between the maternal systems protecting the mother from foreign invasion and the foetal systems protecting the foetus from the maternal onslaught. It is a fight to finish on either side. If the maternal systems win, the foetus gets eliminated. If the foetal systems win, there is a favourable pregnancy outcome. These are two extremes of the spectrum. There are also intermediate results of this fight, and this can result in clinical expressions of what is now called as "obstetric vasculopathies". These include manifestations like intrauterine growth restriction (IUGR), pre-eclampsia, accidental haemorrhage and probably even some of the preterm births. It is now presumed that if theoretically a pregnancy continues indefinitely, eventually the maternal systems will win. The result? At about 55 weeks of pregnancy, every woman will develop pre-eclampsia. In this fight, the free radicals have a big role to play.

The milieu between two cells is called an "intercellular matrix". The interface between the foetus and the mother called the "foetomaternal interface" and is the hotbed where production of ROS occurs. To better understand, one can imagine this foetomaternal interface as site of terrorist training camps. In that comparison, the ROS can then be seen as trainers or dons of terrorists. In that parlance, one can compare lipids as undergoing indoctrination at these camps and get trained as terrorists. This indoctrination process is lipid peroxidation. The foetomaternal interface is the milieu where free radicals bring about a series of changes in the circulating lipid molecules, which subsequently lead to clinical occurrence of pre-eclampsia and other obstetric vasculopathies.

LIPID PEROXIDES: THE AGENTS OF OXIDATIVE STRESS

For understanding the role of oxidative stress in causing pre-eclampsia, one needs to highlight some basics even if it is repetitive. The basic pathology in pre-eclampsia is vasospasm. This vasospasm is generated in the entire maternal vasculature. Free radicals, or ROS themselves, do not have the numbers or the capacity to go through the entire maternal vasculature to cause this vasospasm and the subsequent clinical manifestation of pre-eclampsia. A heavily determined ROS force now needs agents to achieve its aim. It need agents that are more universally distributed, readily available and have the inclination and readiness to get denatured to produce the changes that ROS want from them. Lipid lipoproteins fit this bill perfectly.

Lipoprotein molecules based on their densities are of different groups. These groups, from least dense (largest particles), compared to surrounding water, to most dense (smallest particles), are chylomicrons (ultra-low-density lipoprotein [ULDL] by the overall density naming convention), very-low-density lipoprotein (VLDL), intermediate-density lipoprotein (IDL), low-density lipoprotein (LDL) and high-density lipoprotein (HDL). LDL and VLDL deliver fat molecules to the intercellular matrix and subsequently drive the different changes leading to pre-eclampsia and other obstetric vasculopathies.

The LDL and VLDL are so configured that they tend to go near and sink into the vascular cell linings. It is this propensity that is exploited by the ROS. Early in pregnancy, there is a preponderance of HDLs in the circulation. The density of these molecules is such that they are unable to come close to the cell wall. As a result, the lipid goblets are not able to sink within the intercellular matrix. With advancing normal pregnancy and in abnormal (vasculopathic) early pregnancy, the lipid distribution changes in favour of LDLs and VLDLs. These molecules sink closer to the intercellular matrix (Figures 4.4 and 4.5).

Although density seems to be the principle reason of VLDL and LDL molecules sinking closer to the intercellular matrix, there are other operational reasons, too. One of the important reasons is the quantitative increase in number of these molecules over VLDL as pregnancy advances. One more reason that has remained by and large unstudied is the electronic configuration of these molecules. It seems science has played too much onus on the shoulders of density to bring the VLDL and LDL molecules close to the endothelial lining of the vessel walls. Physical attributes like density, colour, thickness and the like alone are not enough to explain the peculiarity of behaviour of any molecule or particle in nature. There seems to be more to this.

It is also likely that the electronic configuration of these molecules is such that they tend to get attracted to the vessel wall. The extent that this factor operates is a matter of study. Another interesting phenomena needs to be considered in this context: ULDL (chylomicrons) and mid-density lipoproteins (MDLs) are not implicated in the process of lipid peroxidation. The density of ULDL is the least amongst all lipoprotein molecules. MDLs are less than HDL molecules but more than LDL molecules in density. Are they not then ready prey to sinkage in the intercellular matrix? If density was the only factor, why are they not falling a victim to the ROS in the intercellular matrix? This makes one seriously wonder, if there is anything more than the mere physical density of these molecules at play. This is where the electronic configuration of these molecules becomes pertinent. Likely,

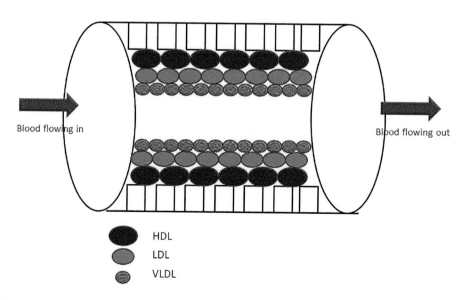

Figure 4.4 Vascular lipid distribution in normal pregnancy (schematic representation). HDL, high-density lipoprotein; LDL, low-density lipoprotein; VLDL, very-low-density lipoprotein.

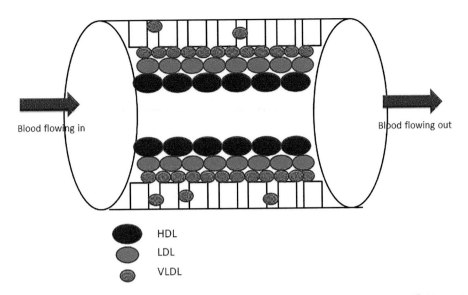

Figure 4.5 Vascular lipid distribution in pregnant women with pre-eclampsia (schematic representation). HDL, high-density lipoprotein; LDL, low-density lipoprotein; VLDL, very-low-density lipoprotein.

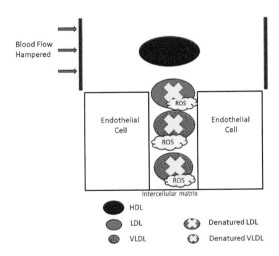

Figure 4.6 Schematic representation of lipid peroxidation on vasospasm. HDL, high-density lipoprotein; LDL, low-density lipoprotein; ROS, reactive oxygen species; VLDL, very-low-density lipoprotein.

VLDL and LDL molecules are electronically also configured in such a way that they get attracted to the endothelial cell wall and intercellular matrix.

On vasospasm, these vulnerabilities are in the intercellular milieu, and the free radicals pounce on them to denature them (Figure 4.6). There is one more change that appears to help this phenomenon of sinkage of lipoproteins into the intercellular

matrix. The slowing of the circulating blood that carries these lipoproteins seems to be a contributing factor. It acts by giving these lipoproteins enough time to get closer to the cell wall and sink within.

It seems like the genetic susceptibility of a woman to developing pre-eclampsia may be playing a small and amorphous role in this. It is now known that the pathophysiology depends not only on the foetal and placental genotype but also on the capability of the maternal system to deal with pregnancy. Genetically, pre-eclampsia is a complex disorder, and despite numerous efforts, no clear mode of inheritance has been established. At least 178 genes have been described concerning pre-eclampsia.[1] The angiotensin-converting enzyme insertion/deletion (ACE I/D) polymorphism is known to affect uteroplacental and umbilical artery blood flows in women with pre-eclampsia. Pre-eclampsia and the haemolysis, elevated liver enzymes, low platelet count, known as the HELLP syndrome, are multiplex genetic diseases.[2] It is suggested that the initial vasospasm, albeit feeble but effective, occurs as a result of this genetic susceptibility of women to pre-eclampsia. These are transient occurrences and occur intermittently. On their own, these vascular impendence tendencies cannot produce significant clinical manifestations.

Nonetheless, they effectively impede the vascular flow to give the time and opportunity to the

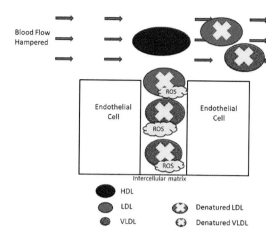

Figure 4.7 On relief of vasospasm denatured lipids flushed into circulation. HDL, high-density lipoprotein; LDL, low-density lipoprotein; ROS, reactive oxygen species; VLDL, very-low-density lipoprotein.

VLDL and LDL molecules to sink to the intercellular matrix. Once they are in the matrix, the ROS are readily available and waiting to denature them, producing lipid peroxidation. As soon as this vascular impedance of transient nature is relieved, the denatured lipid peroxides are flushed into the system during reperfusion (Figure 4.7). Wherever they go, they bring about a tilt in the prostacyclin-thromboxane balance. The balance is tipped in favour of thromboxane producing a vasospasm. It is universally known that the principal and most consistent change universally seen in pre-eclampsia is vasospasm. The genesis of vasospasm is a result of the ROS-lipid peroxidation.

OUR BASIC STUDY

- We carried out a systematic evaluation of pro-oxidants and antioxidants in pre-eclampsia to serve as a basis for our understanding of this disease process.
- It confirmed oxidative stress in normal pregnancy and in pre-eclampsia.
- Natural endogenous antioxidant enzymes activity is enhanced significantly against this oxidative stress to maintain the state of equilibrium in favour of antioxidant defence.
- However, in pre-eclampsia, the antihypertensive therapy showed little change in oxidative stress and like normal pregnancy, the body still maintained increased antioxidant enzyme activity.

- This indicates that though the antihypertensives may reduce the effect of oxidative stress, they cannot stop the cause of it.

This study proved to be the basic first step for us in understanding of this disease process.[3]

LIPID METABOLISM IN NORMAL PREGNANCY AND IN PRE-ECLAMPSIA

Alteration in lipid metabolism leads to dyslipidaemia. Interesting alterations take place in lipid metabolism in normal pregnancy as well as in pre-eclampsia. For understanding anything abnormal, it is imperative to first know the normal. Lipids are carried into circulation primarily as lipoproteins that are composed primarily of free and esterified lipid proteins, which are also known as apolipoprotein and phospholipids.[4] The two main triglyceride carrying lipoproteins are chylomicrons (ULDL) and VLDLs. The two main cholesterol containing lipoproteins are LDLs and HDLs.

Lipids are distributed throughout the body. They are either in the stationary stored form or in the kinetic form. While in stored form, lipids are by and large protected from the process of denaturation. But it is in their kinetic form when being transported that they get vulnerable to denaturation. The entire process of lipid transport, therefore, needs to be understood well if one has to understand the etiological possibilities of pre-eclampsia. Those lipids that are getting transported through the vessel wall are vulnerable to coming close to the intercellular matrix. It is in this matrix that the entire genesis of pre-eclampsia occurs. Stationary lipids stationed in the tissues do not play so much mischief. They are neither prone to any changes at the storage site nor are they likely to undergo the process of pathological destruction and dysfunction there. Therefore, stored lipids are of a limited clinical bearing. It is the circulating lipids that are most susceptible to changes. While in transit, these lipids come in contact with the vascular endothelial wall. Here they undergo the all-important desaturation.

When lipids are the primary players in pre-eclampsia, one can wonder as to why women who are obese with profuse availability of lipids in their body do not suffer from pre-eclampsia consistently? The answer lies in this difference of vulnerability of lipid molecules when stationary and in transit. Labelling obesity is based on the stationary lipids in the body. In clinical practice, young overweight mothers may not necessarily have an increased or altered circulating lipid levels, and until the time that the circulating lipid levels are altered, pre-eclampsia would not manifest. Thus, in clinical practice, one woman who is obese may just register mild pre-eclampsia, whereas a woman who is overweight may have a fulminant form of obstetric vasculopathy. The opposite is also true. Many times in clinical practice, one finds subjects who are lean but progress quickly into pre-eclampsia and full-blown eclampsia. This is again because a subject is labelled as lean based on her weight (dependent on stationary and stored adipose tissue). On the other hand, her pre-eclampsia develops on the basis of circulating lipids.

It is relevant to introduce at this point that statins have been promoted for use in pre-eclampsia increasingly in last decade. Statins are a group of drugs, which act to reduce levels of cholesterol in the blood. Work on use of statins in pregnancy especially in obese subjects began as early as in 1979.[5] However, it is only in the last decade or a few years before that more and more studies were published on their use. Use of these agents in pre-eclampsia, especially its prevention in obese subjects, will be discussed in greater detail in the chapter in prevention of pre-eclampsia.

Neboh et al. showed that in the early weeks and months of pregnancy HDL levels are high in circulation.[6] As pregnancy advances, circulating levels of LDL and VLDL start increasing. The serum lipid levels are significantly higher in all the trimesters of the pregnant woman than in the controls. There was a steady increase in the serum lipid levels with increasing gestational age. A significant positive correlation is observed between the lipid fractions and the different trimesters of pregnancy. For total cholesterol, the HDL ratio is decreased significantly in pregnant women with increasing gestational age. This goes on progressively until term.[6]

Relative insulin resistant states of late pregnancy have a vital role to play in the changes in lipid metabolism all throughout pregnancy. It is well-known that pregnancy is a diabetogenic state.[7] Nevertheless, all pregnancies may not manifest clinical diabetes. This relative insulin resistance progressively increases as pregnancy advances.

As soon as delivery occurs, the relatively altered insulin sensitivity is restored to normal, and the potential diabetogenic state is reversed. Insulin resistance does not clinically manifest as loss of euglycemic states in all pregnant subjects. In most pregnancies, blood sugar levels do not cross their thresholds to be labelled as overt diabetes. However the relative insulin resistance is reflected in circulating insulin levels, which are found to be consistently increasing in pregnancy. Placental growth hormone seems to have an important complementary role in this. Placental growth hormone induces maternal insulin resistance and thereby facilitates the mobilisation of maternal nutrients for foetal growth.[8]

The term "placental growth hormone" says it all; the human growth hormone (GH)/human placental lactogen (hPL) gene family consists of two GHs and three PLs genes. It has an important role in the regulation of maternal and foetal metabolism and the growth and development of the fetus.[9] It is produced by trophoblasts and becomes detectable in maternal serum during the first trimester of pregnancy. Its concentration increases as term approaches and becomes undetectable within 1 hour of delivery. GH has important biological properties, including lipolytic activity.[10] This presumably boosts the release of free fatty acids and glycerol, thereby releasing them into circulation and increasing the substrate for VLDL production.

Oestrogen, the ubiquitous hormone in females, also plays its part in the lipid metabolism in pregnancy. Under the effect of oestrogen, VLDL gets readily released from the liver stores into circulation. The lipolytic activity gets influenced in such a way that with advancing pregnancy VLDL and LDL remain in circulation for a longer time. These changes are taking place to maximise the transfer of maternal essential fatty acids to the foetus. Before the clinical picture of pre-eclampsia becomes obvious, dyslipidaemia has been documented to occur. This dyslipidaemia or disturbed lipid metabolism has been noted as a feature of pre-eclampsia for many decades. However, its importance was not well understood until now.

With the insights into the aetiopathology of obstetric vasculopathies in general and pre-eclampsia, in particular, becoming obvious, the reasons for various changes in lipid metabolism got explained. LDL and VLDL tend to get closer to the vascular endothelium in a dynamic process. Once near the vascular endothelium, these molecules get readily drawn into the intercellular matrix. Here they undergo a process of denaturation. This denaturation is brought about by ROS in a process called "lipid peroxidation". It leads to denaturation of circulating VLDL and LDL. It seems, in nature, the denaturized lipid molecules have hardly any role to play in maintaining a healthy pregnancy. The maternal system needs to supply the so-called "unadulterated" VLDLs and LDLs to the foetomaternal interface for accomplishing many important physiological growth and functions of the foetus. One of the reasons why circulating levels of lipids increase as pregnancy advances is: With a sizable portion of its lipid molecules getting rendered invalid for physiology, the mother increases the levels of unadulterated VLDLs and LDLs. This is not to say that all lipid increase is only for compensation for the mass of lipid molecules that have been denatured. Physiologically, pregnancy also increases the demand for metabolic fuels for foetal growth and development of its associated structures. It has been stated that up to 20% of sterol in the embryo could be derived from maternal placental cholesterol and a possible greater percentage in placentas with hypercholesterolemia.[11] In Smith-Lemli-Opitz syndrome, a congenital defect in cholesterol biosynthesis, foetuses that cannot produce any cholesterol are born with small quantities of serum cholesterol, which confirms that some maternal cholesterol is passed onto the foetus.[11] Foetal needs, therefore, lead to changes in lipid profile during different trimesters of the pregnancy; the additional need for compensation for denaturalisation gets factored in.

However, an interesting phenomenon occurs as soon as the parturient delivers. The circulating increased levels get precipitously reduced as soon as delivery occurs. The healthy lipids that increased are now not needed once the foetus has been delivered. But the harm done by the denaturation process of lipid peroxidation takes the body a longer time to revert to its normal state. Clinically, therefore, one finds that pre-eclampsia does not reverse as dramatically and as consistently as the circulating levels of lipids go back the non-pregnant state.

Changes of pre-eclampsia, including hypertension, may take weeks to reverse. Sometimes, blood pressure may strike the base, giving the signal that the process is over. However in some subjects, after a week or so blood pressure registers a high

again. Sometimes blood pressure may follow a disciplined and graded reversal, and in some other subjects, blood pressure may not show any change for a couple of days or a week and then start declining. Similar behaviour can be seen in other manifestations of pre-eclampsia, including oedema or proteinuria. Even the potentially devastating changes of renal compromise may not follow any pre-decided pattern.

For the changes of pre-eclampsia to occur, an entire orchestra comes into action. Though this orchestra is complex, it is never dysrhythmic. It follows a rhythm. Although dyslipidaemia is just one segment of the entire orchestra in pre-eclampsia, there are a series of other processes also involved. Even if dyslipidaemia reverses, other processes may not. Also, the lipids, essential fatty acids, are needed to maintain their supply to the foetus. Therefore, hyperlipidaemia is maintained when the foetus is still in the uterus. The concurrent process of lipid denaturation, including lipid peroxidation, destroys this all-important supply chain of essential fatty acids to the foetus. To compensate, the mother mobilises more and more essential fatty acids.

But even at lower levels of circulating lipids, the process can still maintain itself. Also, the reversal process does not follow any algorithmic pattern. How much time the vasospasm and reperfusion damage need before the body senses that the process is over is entirely dependent on the innate capacity of the maternal system to reverse or close the process. Even at normal levels of circulating lipids, the process of denaturation can continue.

The fury of late-onset pre-eclampsia is consistently maximum, just before the end of pregnancy. In pre-eclampsia, for example, the blood pressure is highest coupled with oedema and proteinuria just before the delivery. Accidental haemorrhage and its complications are at its peak of activity just before delivery. The process of IUGR occurs unabated and leads to a precipitous decline in foetal fortunes until the time that it delivers.

Serum triglyceride, cholesterol and free fatty acid concentrations decrease sharply in pre-eclampsia and pregnant controls 24–48 hours postpartum.[12,13] However, the fall in triglycerides and cholesterol continues for up to 6 weeks postpartum. The decreasing levels of triglycerides and cholesterol help in sustaining the changes of pre-eclampsia albeit at a lowered intensity. How fast and by what time the levels of triglycerides and cholesterol hit the base of normalcy will depend on the innate maternal systemic responses. They are different and variable for each mother and the same mother in different pregnancies. Accordingly, the changes of pre-eclampsia vary from mother to mother and even in the same mother from pregnancy to pregnancy.

HYPERTRIGLYCERIDEMIA AND PRE-ECLAMPSIA

Fatty acids contribute to endothelial dysfunction in pre-eclampsia by several ways: Free-fatty-acid–mediated endothelial dysfunction facilitates ROS generation.[14] Generation of ROS is one of the most important steps in pre-eclampsia. ROS incite the entire plethora of changes in pre-eclampsia. Yet one big question that always remains in the mind of the scientific investigator is what generates ROS. The answer is free fatty acids.

There is now an established relation amongst hypertriglyceridemia, atherosclerosis and coronary artery disease. In the realms of oxidative stress, monocytes isolated from individuals with hypertriglyceridemia show increased production of superoxides and enhanced binding to endothelial cells.[15] Thus, hypertriglyceridemia generates ROS by first increasing the binding of circulating monocytes to endothelial cells. Thereafter, in quick succession, these monocytes start generating superoxide. For this, hypertriglyceridemia is a consistent precursor and critical event.

The superoxides critically associated with ROS quickly make the latter alive and available in the intercellular matrix. It is then in this intercellular endothelial matrix that the VLDLs and LDLs get ensnared by the ROS to undergo lipid peroxidation. Another important event in this series is the conversion of large LDL particles to small dense LDL particles for the maintenance of the pathology of pre-eclampsia, which needs to be closely understood.

SMALL DENSE LDL PHENOTYPE IN PRE-ECLAMPSIA

The entire LDL family consists of phenotypically different particles. Their difference is based on density, size and chemical structure. It is this phenotype that decides the buoyancy and nature of the LDL particles. Even amongst the cohort of LDL particles, there are two subtypes, the large LDL particles and the small LDL particles. In adult healthy females, the large LDL particles are predominant. They remain buoyant and away from the vessel wall in circulation. They have a definite estrogenic influence. With menopause appearing, these large LDL particles start getting phenotypically metamorphosed to small dense LDL particles. There is also an intermediate subclass of LDL particles not as small and dense as those found in menopausal women and not as large as the LDL particles in other healthy adult non-menopausal females. These are not as buoyant as the large LDL particles. They are found predominantly in adult males. Variation in LDL particle in size and density is under both genetic and non-genetic influence. Amongst non-genetic influence, dietary intake and factors like smoking and coffee drinking also influence these.[16]

In pre-eclampsia, there are distinct metabolic changes that produce hypertriglyceridemia. These generally shift the spectrum of LDL subfractions towards a proportional increase of smaller and denser LDL particles.[4] Small dense LDL particles are relatively depleted of cholesteryl esters and enriched in protein.[17,18] These small dense LDL particles by the innate size and buoyancy as well as their electronic propensity have an increased proteoglycan binding. Galeano et al. suggested as early as in 1998 that small dense LDL might be more atherogenic than normal size LDL because of decreased hepatic clearance by the LDL receptor and enhanced anchoring to LDL receptor-independent binding sites in extrahepatic tissues (e.g., the arterial wall), a process mediated, in part, by cell surface proteoglycans.[19] This proteoglycan binding makes them susceptible to getting closer to the vessel wall and, therefore, the vascular endothelium. Once they come in apposition to or close to the vascular endothelium, they move readily in and out of the intercellular matrix of the vascular endothelium. This is where they undergo the process of LDL lipid peroxidation. Small dense LDL particles have a major influence and contribution in the occurrence of a series of diseased states. Women with higher levels of circulating small dense LDL develop non-insulin-dependent diabetes mellitus more readily. They also had a higher propensity to myocardial infarctions subsequently.

Non-insulin dependent diabetes mellitus and myocardial infarction are usually the diseases of adults and advancing age. This does not hold for pre-eclampsia. Pre-eclampsia does not necessarily occur in elderly pregnant women. In clinical practice, no definite association is found between pre-eclampsia and maternal age. Elderly gravida do seem to tend to develop pre-eclampsia, especially the superimposed pre-eclampsia over under running hypertension. Yet pre-eclampsia does not occur only in the elderly gravida. This goes on to show that pre-eclampsia creates a pathological milieu similar to those in aging. The conversion of large and buoyant LDL particles readily to small dense particles is a direct example of the same. It also goes on to explain the findings of atherosclerosis-like changes at the foetomaternal interface in subjects with pre-eclampsia. This is essentially age-independent and, by and large, reversible in pregnancy.

Interestingly, small dense LDL particles are not only more susceptible to getting drawn towards the vascular endothelium but are also more susceptible to oxidation compared to the large buoyant variety.[20] Proportional increases in small dense LDL with heightened susceptibility to oxidative modification may account for the part of the increased cardiovascular risk in individuals with the small dense LDL phenotype.[21] This may have a genetic basis because of genetic copy number variants in patients with myocardial infarction and hyperlipidemia.[22]

Interestingly, one more characteristic associated with small dense LDL is that these are more susceptible to oxidative degeneration because of decreasing particle size and proportional polyunsaturated fatty acid increase. Concurrently, per each small dense LDL particle, there is a decrease in reducing systems' effectiveness. It, therefore, seems obvious that the pitch for occurrence of pre-eclampsia is foiled competently and decisively by the maternal system.

Compared to their more buoyant and larger LDL particles, small dense LDL particles have a greater capacity to stimulate thromboxane synthesis.[4] They also have an increased capacity to escalate intracellular calcium in smooth muscle cells. The sum total effect of this is an increased propensity to smooth muscle contraction. Thus, the small dense LDL particles lead readily to vasospasm. Interestingly, small dense LDLs have an effect on increasing thromboxane synthesis, but they do not concurrently reduce prostacyclin levels.

This leads to alteration in thromboxane prostacyclin ratio only by affecting one factor of the ratio and not both. The sum total effect of this is that the thromboxane-prostacyclin balance tips in favour of thromboxane. Thromboxane is a well-known vasoconstrictor. So, the net effect is vasoconstriction as found in pre-eclampsia.

The correlation between the size of LDL particle and triglycerides is also interesting. It will have an important bearing in causing pre-eclampsia. The size of LDL particles reduces from the large buoyant variety to the intermediate dense variety as pregnancy progresses from 5–6 weeks to 36 weeks. This subsequently reverts to the prepregnant level nearly completely by 6 weeks postpartum.[4] In an interesting study which proved this gestational progression of LDL diameter was studied prospectively in 10 pregnant non-smoker subjects. It was found that the LDL particle size was negatively correlated with serum levels of triglyceride.[23] This means as the particles became smaller and denser, the triglyceride levels increased.

In physiological parlance, the LDL particles were, therefore, divided into three subtypes. This was based on the size and density of these particles. Particle sizes 1 and 2 were the buoyant variety. Particles of size 3 were the less buoyant variety. It was found that as pregnancy advanced, the size transformed from 1 to 3. In pre-eclampsia, this transformation occurs much faster and much more steeply. It gets reflected in the clinical behaviour of pre-eclampsia. Any pregnant subject becomes more susceptible to pre-eclampsia as pregnancy advances. There are clinical situations wherein pre-eclampsia manifests remote from term. In such pregnancies, this conversion of type 1 and 2 LDL to type 3 LDL occurs much more rapidly. It is critical for the process of aetiopathology of pre-eclampsia that this conversion occurs. If and whenever this conversion occurs, the LDL 3 reaches the intercellular endothelial matrix. As has been made amply clear, LDL particles undergo peroxidation in the matrix to generate and perpetuate pre-eclampsia. It appears that oxidisation of LDL is critical and all important for the aetiopathogenesis of pre-eclampsia.

PLACENTAL LIPID PEROXIDATION

Lipid peroxidation is an important event in the aetiopathology of pre-eclampsia. At this stage, it is relevant to introduce the reader to malondialdehyde

(MDA). MDA is a product of lipid peroxidation. It is increased in placental tissue along with decreased superoxide dismutase (SOD) activity in pre-eclampsia.[24,25] SOD is an important antioxidant. It is present in nearly all living cells exposed to oxygen. Basically, it is a defence molecule. In simple terms, superoxide is produced as a by-product of oxygen metabolism and, if not regulated, causes many types of cell damages. Interestingly several isoforms of SOD exist. This includes cytosolic copper/zinc and mitochondrial manganese.[26] The SOD has a peculiar role in breaking down superoxide. This breaking down renders the superoxide molecule invalid, thereby leading to protection of the foetomaternal interface from oxidative injury. In pre-eclampsia, there is a reduced SOD activity and a consequent increased oxidative stress. Superoxide seems to have a field day in pre-eclampsia. However, superoxide is a vibrant and seemingly determined molecule. It does not accept defeat at the hands of SOD easily. It counter-fights decisively and determinedly. For its part, superoxide tries to alter SOD. It alters two isoforms of SOD, both cytosolic as well as mitochondrial. This renders the activity of SOD paralysed or partly hindered. A partly dysfunctional SOD in the placenta of subjects with pre-eclampsia leads to the unchallenged activity of oxidative free radicals, which subsequently results in lipid peroxidation. Coming back to MDA, then it is one of the most abundant carbonyl products of lipid peroxidation. It is damaging and virulent. MDA has been reported to be mutagenic and carcinogenic.[27] Its importance lies in finding an explanation to the alteration in prostaglandin activity in pre-eclampsia. MDA is a product of lipid peroxidation and prostaglandin biosynthesis. Thus, concurrently while causation of lipid peroxidation; the oxidative process also has a profound effect on prostaglandin metabolism. This explains the link amongst pre-eclampsia, lipid peroxidation and alteration of thromboxane-prostacyclin balance in favour of thromboxane.

Glutathione peroxides have been studied for the lipid peroxidation activity in obstetric vasculopathies, including pre-eclampsia and miscarriages.[28] It has been found that glutathione peroxides are relatively decreased in placenta of women with pre-eclampsia. This change is a marker of an increased lipid peroxidation activity. Interestingly, the chemical inhibition of placental glutathione peroxides results in release of hydroperoxides and an increase in the placental thromboxane-to-prostacyclin output ratio.[29] The relative deficiency of glutathione peroxides in placenta of women with pre-eclampsia occurs in conjunction with increase tissue production of lipid hydroperoxides and thromboxane A_2.[29] These observations are important. The process of lipid peroxidation and flushing of the lipid peroxides into circulation provides an important link with alteration in the prostacyclin-to-thromboxane ratio in favour of thromboxane. Lipid peroxides are therefore critical in the foundation for generating changes that lead to vasospasm – the hallmark pathological event of pre-eclampsia. Demonstration of decreased prostacyclin production or the increased thromboxane production in conjunction with increased lipid peroxidation establishes the link between the two. It, therefore, seems that the entire oxidative process through nearly all its by-products and markers alter the prostaglandin metabolism.

Once this link is established, it becomes easy to understand the plethora of clinical manifestations that occur in pre-eclampsia in particular and obstetric vasculopathies in general. The basic pathology in all obstetric vasculopathies is vasospasm. One can easily understand the fact that even if one of the factors of any ratio is altered, the result is altered as well. This means that if prostacyclin production decreases, thromboxane supervenes to produce a tilt in balance towards vasospasm. Alternatively, if thromboxane production is singularly increased, so will the resultant manifestation. But in pre-eclampsia, the alteration that occurs is thorough. Both the components of the ratio get altered. This makes the pathology more profound and devastating.

Glutathione peroxidase reduction in pre-eclampsia is in conjunction with increased thromboxane A_2 production. Lipid hydroperoxides, on the other hand, inhibit prostacyclin syntheses activity. While lipid hydroperoxides inhibit the prostacyclin syntheses activity, they simultaneously also stimulate the cyclooxygenase component of prostaglandin-H synthase. Cyclooxygenase is an important molecule to propagate the conversion of arachidonic acid to the cycle of prostaglandins. By stimulation of cyclooxygenase activity, lipid hydroperoxides ensure that the entire prostaglandin production cycle also gets maintained or perpetuated. This is a critical phenomenon. Merely a single or some episodic alteration in the thromboxane-to-prostacyclin ratio would not suffice to bring about a perpetuated series of changes in preeclampsia. There has to be a system in place which perpetuates the cycle. By influencing the cyclooxygenase production, oxidative stress ensures that the pathology gets perpetuated.

TRANSITION METALS IN LIPID PEROXIDATION

Lipid peroxidation is essentially oxidative deterioration of polyunsaturated fatty acids. It is interesting to find that the lipid peroxidation process has an important role for transition metals, including iron for its amplification.[30] As the first step when the free radical (ROS) comes in contact with the lipid molecules that are susceptible (poly unsaturated fatty acids [PUFA]), they extract methylene hydrogen from unsaturated fatty acids (LH) forming a lipid radical (L^+). This lipid radical reacts with molecular oxygen to form a lipid peroxyl radical (LOO^+). This LOO^* attacks another molecule of LH (unsaturated lipid) to enter a chain. LH gets attacked by LOO^* to produce another LOO^*, which in turn attacks another LH and, thereby, generates one wheel of the vicious circle (Figure 4.8).

Concurrently, attempts are made to magnify or amplify the LOO^* formation. Thus, one section of this vicious circle starts interacting with transition metals like Fe^*, which are dislocated from the intracellular compartments. These transition metals undergo a conversion while amplifying the catalytic conversion of LH to LOO^* and LO^*. Thus, smaller amount of peroxidised lipid radicals is generated by the direct attack of ROS on PUFA, which then enters the same vicious cycle of denaturing LH – unsaturated fatty acids. The same process concurrently gets amplified in its parallel arm when the transition metals like Fe^* get involved in the process.

Although this entire process of lipid peroxidation is on at the intercellular matrix of the vessel wall, the circulation of blood has been relatively impeded. In that short period of vasospasm followed by reperfusion, this process gets completed. Also, the neutralisation of the free radicals by maternal and trophoblastic reducing systems is taking place concurrently. This means that while the destructive or morbidity causing the process of free radical generation and lipid peroxidation is on, the activity of healing by reducing systems is also on. These reducing systems not only stop at neutralising the free radicals but also serve as scavengers eliminating them from the system. In most situations of a healthy pregnancy, the process of neutralisation and elimination by reducing systems overwhelms the destructive systems. This clinically results in a healthy live birth. If however, the destructive process gets an upper hand and overwhelms, the reducing systems obstetric vasculopathies, including pre-eclampsia, result.

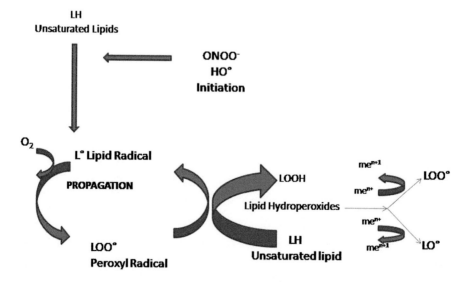

Figure 4.8 Transition of metals. HO•, hydroxyl radical; L•, lipid radical; LH, lipid hydroxyl radical (unsaturated lipids); LO•, lipid alkoxylradical; LOO•, lipid peroxyl radical; LOOH, lipid hydroperoxides; Me, transition metal; O_2, oxygen; ONOO−, peroxynitrite (sometimes called peroxonitrite) radical.

The process of lipid peroxidation in particular and that of oxidative stress is not always a disease-causing process. There are quite a few processes of health that are dependent on free radicals and lipid peroxidation as has been hinted in previous sections. The classic example of a process that gets propagated thus is the process of activation of the cyclooxygenase component of prostaglandin-H (PGH) synthase, which requires the presence of lipid hydroperoxides.[31]

CLINICAL MANIFESTATIONS

Once it is understood why vasospasm occurs in pre-eclampsia, it will be easy to explain different clinical features and complications of pre-eclampsia. Vascular impedance from vasospasm throughout the maternal vasculature makes the maternal system sense difficulty in critical blood flow through the maternal vascular bed. Once the mother's body senses that it is unable to maintain effective blood supply to vital systems, it starts forcing the blood through her vascular channels. This increase in the force of blood through the vessels is clinically manifested as hypertension and pre-eclampsia.

Intermittent vasospasm and reperfusion denude the vessels of proper protection of its walls. To what extent is the vasa-vasorum involved in this is difficult to study. However, the damage to the vessel walls could be a result of both direct injuries as well as dysfunctional vasa-vasorum. The damaged vessel walls can withstand the vasospasm. However, when this spasm is relieved, the vessel walls give way. Destroyed integrity of the vessels leads to leakage of blood at the foetomaternal interface, resulting in a known complication of pre-eclampsia, accidental haemorrhage.

REPERFUSION

The pathognomonic lesion in pre-eclampsia is vasospasm. Although this has been the most conspicuous change to the examining eye of the pathologist, in actuality it is not the vasospasm that produces the clinical effects. It is in fact the reperfusion damage. Reperfusion damage is intense. Associates of our group carried out an interesting animal experiment about two decades ago.[32] Under strict rules and standards needed and all necessary permissions obtained that were needed at that time, for any such experiment, they passed a wire and blocked the circulation through the internal carotid

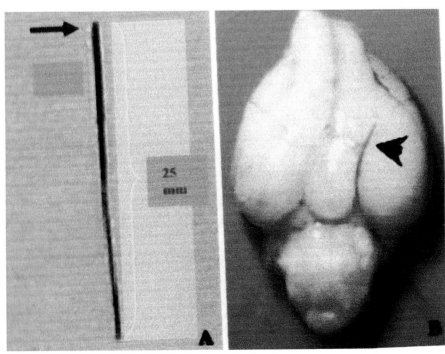

Figure 4.9 Carotid artery block and brain of experimental animal.

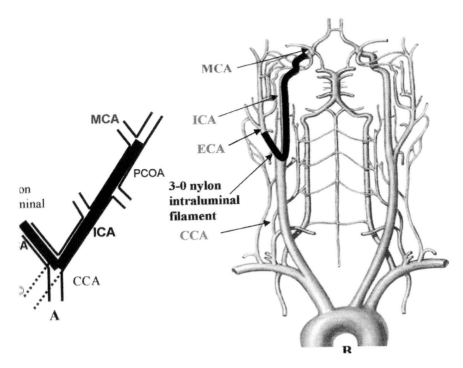

Figure 4.10 Schematic diagram of carotid circulation and block.

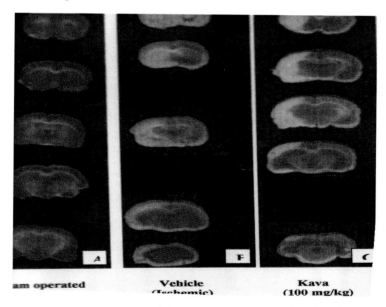

Figure 4.11 Post-reperfusion damage of the experimental brain. A: Unaffected brain in blocked arteries but no reperfusion, B: Brains after removal of the block on reperfusion showing ischemic injury, and C: Antioxidant Kava unable to prevent the ischemic injury on reperfusion.

of experimental dogs unilaterally (Figures 4.9 and 4.10). The other side was perfusing the brain of the dogs normally. While this block continued, no damage occurred. As soon as the block was removed, perfusion was re-established. Under the effect of this reperfusion, profound injuries occurred to the canine brain. As the next step, they were now perfused with a strong antioxidant (Kava). However, this antioxidant could at best only partly neutralise the reperfusion damage (Figure 4.11).

The result of this experiment has interesting insight into the process of reperfusion damage. While it ascertains that it is not the vasospasm but the reperfusion that causes harm, it also highlights a bigger challenge. This challenge is related to the limitation of the reducing substances in preventing or reversing the reperfusion damage.

Even in clinical practice, it is well-known that reducing substances, or antioxidants as they are called, are unable to completely ameliorate or prevent pre-eclampsia. They can, at best, limit their damage. However, what damage will be limited and to what extent is never predictable. It depends on the maternal systems undergoing the damage of reperfusion and the adequacy of antioxidants for that tissue or body to counteract the oxidative stress resulting in the complications of pre-eclampsia.

INNATE MATERNAL REDUCING SYSTEMS

Metaphorically, pregnancy has been described as a boxing ring to make the understanding of the graft-host reactions easier. In this ring, there is a perpetual fight between the foetal survival systems and maternal rejection systems. The mother bears the brunt of the foetal graft in the form of a series of changes, resulting from the complex immunology and oxidative stress interplay. Concurrently, her system also generates a series of protective systems. This can well be compared with boxers in the ring who hits the opponent and at the same time also protects themselves. Here the opponent is the foreign foetal system.

Thankfully, the maternal protective systems are much more powerful and efficient. As a result, clinical manifestations of any of the obstetric vasculopathies, including pre-eclampsia, do not occur. As soon free radicals are generated, reducing radicals also get generated in the mother. Most of the time, maternal reducing systems are powerful enough to protect the host (mother) efficiently. It will be of interest to know that these protective systems cannot protect for infinite duration of time. It is estimated that if the pregnancy continues for an unlimited period, theoretically, by 55 weeks, every pregnancy will have clinical manifestations of pre-eclampsia.

In every pregnancy, some amount of sinkage of VLDLs and LDLs is bound to occur. This is the innate tendency of these molecules to seek the intercellular matrix. Once in the matrix, the free radicals when neutralised by maternal reducing systems would not be enough to peroxidase the lipid molecules. The lipids that may get peroxidised are in a small amount. Although they reach circulation, they do produce vasospasm. However, at the level of the tissues, the protective guards are present. These are tissue-reducing systems, and they completely overwhelm the peroxidised lipid molecules, rendering them incapable of producing much harm. Once neutralised, the peroxidised lipids are not in a position to generate the vasospasm-reperfusion-vasospasm damage chain.

Maternal vasculature during pregnancy has a bias towards maintaining the calibre of the vessels and, thereby, effective circulation in the tissues and organs. The thromboxane-prostacyclin balance tilts in favour of prostacyclin, causing an effective and competent circulation of the organs and tissues. During pregnancy, maternal blood tends to be hypercoagulable and tends to clot easily. This is a protective change that occurs to counteract the blood loss that readily occurs in a pregnant woman most during labour. Despite the blood being hypercoagulable, the perfusion of the maternal system is excellently maintained. This is a little paradoxical but understandable. The hypercoagulable state, in an intact maternal vascular system, is not causing any harm. It also does not clog up the maternal vascular bed.

In the eventuality of failure of maternal protective reducing systems, devastation follows. It is apparent that pre-eclampsia occurs not as a result of one of the following but as a result of all of these:

- Genetic interplay,
- Immune maladaptation,
- Imbalance between free oxygen radicals and reducing systems (i.e., scavengers) in favour of the former) and
- Placental ischemia.

All four were originally proposed as theories to explain occurrence of pre-eclampsia. Deep insights into the entire basket of pathologies of obstetric vasculopathies (including pre-eclampsia) reveal that all four of them are acting, in combination, to produce these conditions.

Decreased expression of reducing systems thioredoxin and glutaredoxin in placentae from pregnancies with pre-eclampsia has been documented.[33]

It was found that maternal expression of reducing systems was significantly reduced in pre-eclampsia. This is interesting. It now becomes apparent that the maternal generation of free radicals and resultant perpetuation of the spasm-reperfusion-spasm cycle is pronounced in pre-eclampsia. Concurrently, the maternal production of reducing systems gets reduced. The free radicals, generated in huge and increasing amounts, overwhelm the maternal reducing systems. At the same time, the maternal reducing system generation is also greatly reduced. Thus, increase in the generation of ROS is perpetuated by reduced production of reducing systems, which together combine to produce pre-eclampsia.

In non-diseased states, there is a vital role for reducing systems at the level of the foetomaternal interface. Efficient reducing systems have been identified on the trophoblasts. The origin of this could be the trophoblast itself. The trophoblasts have been known to possess an inborn resistance to the maternal destructive process. Just as the trophoblastic resilience to maternal rejection is efficient so is their ability to generate protective systems. By generation of reducing systems on their surface, trophoblasts protect the pregnancy from maternal oxidative stress distribution.

Proteins thiol-disulphide oxidoreductases such as thioredoxin, glutaredoxin and protein disulphide isomerase have been found to eliminate ROS. Protein thiol-disulphide oxidoreductases, therefore, have an important role in pre-eclampsia.[33] Results from this and similar studies indicate that pre-eclamptic pregnancies were exposed to oxidative stress and the protein thiol-disulphide oxidoreductases were adaptively induced for protection in pre-eclamptic placentae.[4]

A diverse array of cellular and extracellular fluid reducing systems has evolved to control and compartmentalise but not necessarily eliminate the production of ROS.[4] Reducing systems examined in normal and pre-eclamptic pregnancies include the enzymatic reducing systems (i.e., SOD catalase and glutathione peroxidase) and transition metal-binding proteins (i.e., transferrin, ceruloplasmin and ferritin). These are also low molecular mass that serve as scavengers, which directly, primarily and exclusively target free radical and protects in the extracellular compartment.[4] These include water-soluble forms of ascorbate, glutathione and protein thiols and uric acid. They also include lipoprotein and membrane soluble forms including OC-tocopherol (vitamin D).[34]

THE FAMILY OF FREE RADICALS

Most free radicals fall in the category of ROS and superoxide anion radical (O_2^+) and also reactive oxygen derivatives that do not contain unpaired electrons, such as hydrogen peroxide (H_2O_2), hypochlorous acid (HOCL) and peroxynitrite anion (ONOO−).[4] Systems altered to generate ROS during post-ischemic reperfusion include mitochondrial respiration, neutrophil nicotinamide adenine dinucleotide phosphate (NADPH) oxidase, xanthine oxidase and cyclooxygenase.[4] On similar lines, one animal experiment showed exogenous melatonin protects against ischemia/reperfusion-induced oxidative damage to mitochondria in rat placenta, emboldening these researchers to suggest that melatonin could be useful in treating pre-eclampsia.[35] Interestingly iron delocalized from its normal intracellular compartments during ischemic damage will also promote ROS generation upon reoxygenation and reperfusion.

When this process is confined to the foetomaternal interface, it results in IUGR. When it gets expanded to the entire maternal vasculature, it results in pre-eclampsia clinically. The poverty of quality placentation makes placental sinus walls susceptible to ischemic damage, causing it to be rendered asunder and resulting in clinical abruptio placenta or accidental haemorrhage.

In the initial understanding of obstetric vasculopathy, it was thought that maternal vasospasm of pre-eclampsia extends as vasospasm in the placenta causing IUGR. However, with this complex interplay becoming obvious, it is now clear that pre-eclampsia and IUGR do not share the cause-and-effect relationship. They are two manifestations of the same pathophysiology. To make it simple: Pre-eclampsia and IUGR do not have a mother (pre-eclampsia) to daughter (IUGR) relationship. They have a sister-sister relationship, both resulting from the same pathophysiology at different locales.

VASCULAR ENDOTHELIUM AND OXIDATIVE STRESS

Vascular endothelium pays the price of its continuous exposure to blood. Besides the many contents of blood that brush past the vessel wall, the active components leave great effects on the vascular endothelial lining. Whereas circulating lipids have a positive effect on the cell wall, the state of dyslipidaemia produces a diseased state or endothelial cell dysfunction. VLDL and LDL particles can walk in and out of the intercellular matrix because of their cell size and their electronic configuration. This makes them susceptible to denaturation by cell-derived oxidative particles. To protect them, the intercellular matrix has reducing systems which protect these lipids.

Two events provided some leads for the scientists in understanding the aetiopathology of pre-eclampsia. One of them is neutrophil activation, suggesting a process of inflammation, and the other is the process of lipid peroxidation. Neutrophil activation occurs with the process of obstetric vasculopathy, including pre-eclampsia, and resolves with delivery irrespective of the obstetric outcome. On the other hand, lipid peroxidation is elevated before and continues even for some time after delivery. In reality, lipid peroxidation may go on in the body at a much-attenuated level throughout life, indicating the possibility of some role played by the same in the aging process of atherosclerosis.

It appears that in pre-eclampsia the process of neutrophil activation seems to get much more profound in the presence of uninhibited lipid peroxidation. This prompted some workers to suggest that the entire process of obstetric vasculopathy is an inflammatory response. One study measured alpha-1 antitrypsin (AAT), an anti-protease, anti-inflammatory, and tissue-protective molecule in pre-eclampsia.[36] This study was done on the basis of a thinking that unopposed inflammation might be contributing to pre-eclampsia. The AAT levels were studied to know whether the levels of this anti-inflammatory molecule in pre-eclampsia were lower than normal. It was found that there was an association between lower AAT levels and severe pre-eclampsia during pregnancy. But it was wisely concluded that further studies are required to identify the mechanism behind the association and the possibility of safe AAT augmentation for individuals with insufficient circulating AAT.[36] Nevertheless, it is clear that anti-inflammatory agents fail to stem pre-eclampsia. The inflammatory process may be at the most a side process with a minimal modifying role. A reference will once again be made to this inflammation process while the possible role

of nitric oxide will be examined in aetiology of pre-eclampsia in subsequent pages.

INEFFICIENT SECOND WAVE OF TROPHOBLASTIC INVASION

Trophoblasts seem to be a specialized cell lining. At the first step or first wave, they have a critical anchoring role. The first wave of trophoblastic invasion anchors the placenta with the maternal surface. This occurs early in pregnancy. It may be as early as 1 week and may get completed by the fourth week of pregnancy. Near simultaneously, another amazing phenomenon is occurring: This is the second wave of trophoblastic invasion. The second wave of trophoblastic invasion has an extremely specialised function. It is confined to the maternal spiral arterioles in the uterine vasculature. These trophoblasts mould and modify the spiral arterioles in such a way that the latter get shielded off from maternal circulation. As a result, circulating compounds in the maternal circulation, which can alter the calibre of the vessels, are rendered ineffective to generate this altering effect on foetal vasculature. At the same time, they also destroy the muscular wall of the spiral arterioles. This makes the foetoplacental interface, a low-resistance pool of circulation. It seems that there may be Hypoxia Inducible Factor (HIF) that directly alters the cellular responses to low oxygen, which in turn influences the trophoblast lineage commitment and thereby promotes the development of the invasive trophoblast lineage.[37]

Once shielded from the maternal influence, the foetomaternal vascular pool becomes a near-autonomous circulation system. It also has a low impedance flow, thereby leading to a specialised efficient gushing blood pool. Whereas the second wave of trophoblastic invasion has a critical role in the creation of this autonomous circulation pool, inefficient or failed second wave leads to a wide array of clinical effects, including pre-eclampsia.

Although the hypoxic environment promotes trophoblastic generation and growth, beyond a certain point, it plays a pathological role. It, therefore, has a dual purpose: of health when under control, but once uncontrolled, an impediment to trophoblastic invasion. This impediment sets the stage and sows the seeds for obstetric vasculopathies, including pre-eclampsia. Unmoulded spiral arterioles, plugged by the partly failed second wave of trophoblastic invasion, become the hotbed for a generation of free radicals. Also, as a direct effect of this hypoxia is that the generation of protective reducing systems is reduced both in amount as and competence. Though the entire phenomenon of hypoxia generation of ROS and subsequent lipid peroxidation has a critical role to play, it may not be the only aetiopathological phenomenon for the cause of pre-eclampsia. One more phenomenon that may have some modifying role in pre-eclampsia is the generation of vascular endothelial growth factors.

PRODUCTION OF VASCULAR ENDOTHELIAL GROWTH FACTORS

Vascular Endothelial Growth Factors (VEGFs) are a subfamily of growth factors derived from platelets or platelet-derived growth factors. They are known to be decreased in pre-eclampsia.[38] VEGF production and behaviour seems to have an interesting role in the causation pathology of pre-eclampsia. The VEGF are a signal protein produced by cells at different locations of the body. Their essential role is to stimulate formation of new vessels and maintain these vessels functionally and structurally (vasculogenesis and angiogenesis). Vasculogenesis involves de novo formation of embryonic circulatory systems, and angiogenesis means growth and renovation of already existing vascular system. They have a role in health as well as in disease. The VEGF have

a big role in supporting embryonic development.[39] They are believed to have a critical role in the aetiology of endometriosis.[40]

Though there are many known types of VEGF, the activity of VEGF-A was identified first. Before other types of VEGF were discovered, VEGF-A was only known and therefore was named simply VEGF. However later on other types of VEGF got identified and were classified as VEGF-A, B, and so on. All types of VEGF family members act by binding on cell surfaces to receptors. In cases of VEGF, there are tyrosine kinase receptors (VEGFRs) on the cell surface. VEGF bind to VEGFRs to dimerize them. This leads to activation through the process of transphosphorylation. In pregnancy, there has been a high and positive correlation between VEGF and hormones, reflecting placental function like human chorionic gonadotropin (HCG) and progesterone. VEGF production may be increased by these two placental hormones, having a positive effect on trophoblast development. The functions of different VEGF are summarized in Table 4.1.

When VEGF were studied during the menstrual cycle, it was found that VEGF activity in the form of expression and action was greatly increased in decidual cells of early pregnancy. During the menstrual cycle, VEGF activity becomes most pronounced when progesterone is added to the oestrogen in the secretory phase of the endometrium. In short, VEGF and VEGFRs play an important role in implantation and maintenance of normal pregnancy. With

Table 4.1 VEGF type specific functions

Type	Function
VEGF-A	• Angiogenesis • Increased migration of endothelial cells • Increased mitosis of endothelial cells • Increased methane monooxygenase activity • Increased Avβ3 activity • Creation of blood vessel lumen • Creates fenestrations • Chemotactic for macrophages and granulocytes • Vasodilatation (indirectly by NO release)
VEGF-B	Embryonic angiogenesis
VEGF-C	Lymphangiogenesis
VEGF-D	Needed for the development of lymphatic vasculature surrounding lung bronchioles
PlGF	Important for vasculogenesis, also needed for angiogenesis during ischaemia, inflammation, wound healing and cancer.

Abbreviations: NO, nitric oxide; PlGF, placental growth factor; VEGF, vascular endothelial growth factors.

such an interesting role played, scientists wondered if the estimation of VEGF levels may be used for predicting pre-eclampsia and other obstetric vasculopathies. For this, a comparison of their levels was done between placenta of obstetric vasculopathies, like pre-eclampsia and IUGR, and placenta from a normal pregnancy. Some studies found increased expression of VEGF in pre-eclampsia,[41,42] whereas others found that free VEGF are not competent to predict the development of pre-eclampsia.[43] It has also been found that the expression of the new growth factor endocrine gland-derived vascular endothelial growth factor (EG-VEGF) is high in early pregnancy but falls after 11 weeks, suggesting an essential role for this factor in early pregnancy.[44]

NITRIC OXIDE IN PRE-ECLAMPSIA

Nitric oxide (NO) is one of the most potent vasodilators in the human body. It was once marvelled as the molecule of the century and attempts were made to identify its role in conditions of human health and disease. However, in human pregnancy NO seems to have a limited compensatory role. Its role is restricted to one of the several attempts made by the foetomaternal vascular interface to prevent reperfusion damage. This is in contrast to many other systems, tissues and organs of the body in which NO is supposed to promote the health of these structures and not merely prevent destruction by disease processes. It is now clear that reperfusion damage occurs by liberation of a series of vasoconstrictive and vasospasmic elements in the system. NO seems to have a role in reversing this vasospasm. In these endothelial constitutive nitric oxide synthase (ecNOS) gives vital leads.

This enzyme, ecNOS, is found in the basic constitution of the endothelium. It generates NO by catalytic action. In the human placenta, NO synthesis and generation is not innate but as a reaction or result to reperfusion. It means that NO appears at foetomaternal interface only as a response to vasospasm and subsequent reperfusion. This is in contrast to some tissue and organ cell lines where NO is present autonomously on its own. It does not appear as a reaction or in response to phenomenon of vasospasm. In tissues and organs where NO is innately present, it is believed that its role is in promoting the health of these body constituents. But at the foetomaternal interface, NO has a responsive role. Its role is to reverse the harm or

injury or, at best, limit an injury. Therefore, it probably does not have so much significance in human pregnancy. Thus, the molecule of the century, NO, may not be so consistently exalted for human pregnancy. It has been found that in pre-eclampsia, the messenger RNA (mRNA) expression of ecNOS is significantly increased.[45] This reflects the compensatory and protective responsiveness to vascular reperfusion. The expression of mRNA for generating ecNOS occurs only after the process of vasospasm and reperfusion sets in. Therefore, increased generation of NO seems to be on adaptive response of the foetomaternal vasculature to poor perfusion in pre-eclampsia.

It is by now apparent that this entire process of obstetric vasculopathy has some modulator bearing on it by the process of inflammation. It has been found that when human placental extract is infiltrated in the thighs of rats, there was a distinct attenuation of inflammatory response.[46] In these experimental locations, it was also found that besides other factors, NO synthesis was significantly reduced. This observation requires careful understanding. Placental tissue in itself not only does not need the production of NO in the absence of pre-eclampsia, but it positively reduces the generation of nitric oxide (NO). It is, therefore, possible that in the absence of reperfusion damage, the placenta does not need NO. Not only does it not need NO, but it also ensures a reduction in the generation of NO in situations where there is no reperfusion damage. Therefore, if the human foetomaternal interface senses that the milieu is conducive to a healthy pregnancy, NO is dispensed with.

NITRIC OXIDE AND ENDOTHELIAL CELLS

Leads from some in vivo and in vitro studies have given some interesting insights into the possible role of NO in pre-eclampsia. These insights are indirect and circumstantial but nevertheless important. Nitric oxide synthase (NOS) is an enzyme that elaborates NO. Increased activity levels of NOS leads to increased levels of NO in the body. There are different physiological processes in the body which upregulate this enzyme. With the upregulation of NOS, NO levels increase. Using this background one needs to understand the role of NO in pre-eclampsia. It has been found that endothelial cells exposed to plasma of pregnant women with pre-eclampsia in vitro increase the levels of NO. This is intriguing as it is in total contrast to the results of in vitro studies wherein endothelial cells showed an increase in NO levels when exposed to plasma of pregnant women with pre-eclampsia compared with NO levels released by endothelial cells exposed to plasma of pregnant women without pre-eclampsia.[47,48]

The explanation for these paradoxical observations is complex but important. It has demonstrated that the LDL component of plasma is responsible for NO release from the endothelium. Further research in this matter showed that lysophosphotidyl choline, a component of an LDL denatured through the oxidative process, upregulated NOS. NOS is the enzyme that releases the NO. This NO is then expected to neutralise the oxidized lipid peroxides.[49,50] It seems that in their innate form in the body, NO gets quickly used up in neutralising the oxidised LDL. However, in vitro, the endothelium is exposed to a much-diluted plasma. The plasma from pregnant women with pre-eclampsia used to react against the endothelial cells is diluted (2%).[51] In the diluted plasma, the oxidised LDL also gets diluted. The effect of this is the endothelial cells produce NO, and it remains unused for a longer time. This causes a rise in levels in vitro when exposed to plasma of pregnant women with pre-eclampsia.

One more important conclusion that emerges from these studies also needs to be understood and appreciated. While plasma from pregnant women with pre-eclampsia showed a rise in NO released from the endothelium, no such rise was shown by the endothelial cells when exposed to the plasma of pregnant women without pre-eclampsia. This difference is apparently in LDL. Whereas LDL is present in both plasma is similar (though diluted) in strength, the LDL of the pregnant women with pre-eclampsia caused a rise in NO levels from the endothelial cells. The same LDL did not cause any rise when from pregnant women without pre-eclampsia. This proves that both LDLs are seemingly making the difference. The difference in LDLs is not in the concentration of its particles. This difference is principally like these LDL molecules. The LDLs from pregnant women with pre-eclampsia are oxidised LDLs. On the other hand, in plasma from pregnant women without pre-eclampsia, no such denaturation occurs. Thus, LDL from pregnant women with pre-eclampsia is different from LDL from pregnant women without pre-eclampsia. While underlining

the difference like LDLs from two groups, one more basic fact gets proven through these observations: Denatured LDLs (peroxidised LDLs) are principal players in the causation of obstetric vasculopathy.

PLACENTAL ATHEROSIS IN PRE-ECLAMPSIA

In some studies, the phenomenon of placental atherosis has been demonstrated. This is similar to aging atherosis in human beings.[52] It led to speculation that obstetric vasculopathy results from the process of atherosis at the foetomaternal interface. The pathologic lesions of the decidual arterioles bear a striking resemblance to the atherotic lesions of coronary arteries. Both show fibrinoid necrosis of the vessel wall, aggregation of platelets and accumulation of lipid-laden macrophages. It is not specific to pre-eclampsia. It is also demonstrated in other obstetric vasculopathies like IUGR.[52] Under light microscopy, these changes were limited to registering an excess of villous cytotrophoblasts. But under the electron microscopy, these placentae showed much more profound changes. There was villous cytotrophoblastic hyperplasia, focal syncytial necrosis, microvillus abnormalities, reduced syncytial secretory activity, irregular thickening of the trophoblastic basement membrane and the presence of small foetal vessels in the villi.[4]

These changes are due to the result of placental ischemia. This ischaemia was the key aetiological factor for the proponents of placental ischemia theory in causing pre-eclampsia. But a series of observations have shown that ischaemia is just a part of the chain of events that end in pre-eclampsia.

Whilst the basic oxidative stress process is so well established in causing pre-eclampsia, the oxidised products are not demonstrated in maternal vasculature. This is important because it proves that the atheromatous process is confined to the foetomaternal interface. It is, therefore, also clear that the origin of all obstetric vasculopathies occurs at this interface. The maternal vasculature gets secondarily and most of the times reversibly involved.

EXTRACELLULAR REDUCING SYSTEMS

Having had understood the oxidative stress basis of the aetiopathology of pre-eclampsia, it will now be interesting to study the body reaction to this destructive process. In any live system, whenever a destructive potential is activated, the body immediately activates healing or neutralising systems. A classic example of this is the healing and reparative processes in wounds and incisions. As soon as a cut is made on any live human organ or tissue, including the skin, at that moment, the fibroblasts start proliferating to promote healing of that wound. Though clinically the primary healing of any wound may occur within 72–96 hours, it is well-known that the first outpour of fibroblasts occurs the moment the injury occurs. The body not only activates mechanisms to control blood loss in an injury (platelets and coagulation cascade activation), but it also activates mechanisms to heal concurrently. Similarly as soon as oxidative denaturation begins, extracellular reducing systems start their process of neutralising the oxidative injury. As soon as the oxidative injury begins, the extracellular reducing systems start getting liberated in the intercellular matrix. They react with the oxidising free radicals. In actuality, they react much faster with the free radicals than the free radicals react with maternal tissues. Therefore, in most instances, the reducing systems win. They neutralise oxidative injuries or successfully prevent these injuries from occurring. As a result in most instances, the clinical manifestation of pre-eclampsia does not occur.

Whether a molecule acts as an oxidising substance or a reducing system in any given interaction can often be predicted from tables of standard 1-electron reduction potentials.[53] For example, $\alpha(x)$-tocopherol (X-TOH) slows lipid peroxidation by scavenging lipid peroxyl radicals (LOO$^{•}$).[54] This breaks the peroxidation chain: LOO$^{•}$+ X-TOH + X-TOO$^{•}$. Lipid peroxyl radicals get peroxidised in this reaction to LOOH where the reductant X-TOH provides the hydroxyl radical to complete the reaction. But the radical so formed XTOO$^{•}$ is any day less reactive than the initial peroxyl radical LOO$^{•}$.[55]

This is just one example of a successful neutralization of oxidising reactions. A series of such reducing systems are innately active in the extracellular matrix working efficiently and maintaining the health of a pregnant woman. However, when the oxidative reactants are more powerful, numerous and competent, the maternal reducing systems get overwhelmed. Once overwhelmed, the maternal extracellular reducing systems are unable to stem the oxidative process in the extracellular matrix. Unchecked, the oxidative radicals and the oxidative process successfully overwhelm the lipid moieties that are walking in and out of the matrix, and the basic aetiopathology of pre-eclampsia gets rolling.

One classic example of a competent extracellular reducing system is ascorbic acid. In the reaction described in the preceding paragraph, ascorbate sustains the continuous supply and regeneration of Xα-TOH by reducing tocopherol radicals in the membranes and lipoproteins at the water lipid interface. Just as the ROS use the peroxidised lipids to fan out in the foetomaternal interface in particular and in the entire maternal system in general, so do the reducing systems fan out their protection net in the same locations. The reductant change generated by the ascorbate on Xα-TOH is one such classic example. In the maternal systems, ascorbate is a super reducing system. There are many other reducing systems working equally competently.

URIC ACID: THE POWERHOUSE REDUCTANT

Uric acid has been known to play a cardinal role in disease states. Like ascorbic acid, uric acid, or urate, is one of the most powerful extracellular reducing systems in the body. It is operational in all human bodies consistently thwarting and neutralising the disease-producing tendencies of oxidative reactions. Interestingly, average clinicians include the estimation of uric acid in the routine list of laboratory investigations list that they request in pre-eclampsia. Uric acid levels are, therefore, most consistently requested in pre-eclampsia and eclampsia. However, a single value of uric acid estimate does not contribute much in assisting the clinician for any form of decision making. Uric acid behaves like a policeman when it comes to neutralising the oxidative reaction. One can understand the role of these reductants better if we visit the policeman-to-riot model.

Policeman-to-riot model to understand uric acid

If for the sake of understanding, one assumes that oxidative stress is a riot and free radicals are rioters, then reducing systems are policemen mobilised by the mother to quell these riots. If the rioters are more vitriolic or more numerous, the riots go uncontrolled and great destruction can ensue. However, if the policemen are competently armed or are more in number, the riots are quelled from spreading or nipped from the bud. When a clinician requests a single estimation of uric acid, it is similar to seeing some policemen at one instance. It only gives an idea that some riots may be happening. It does not give any further information. Super-normal levels of uric acid at any one given instance provide the information that the oxidative riot may be on, and so the group of policemen (uric acid) is present on duty.

However, when one repeats uric acid estimation in any subject in whom the process of pre-eclampsia has manifested clinically, then there are three possibilities:

1. Uric acid levels may not be much different than those values before three weeks. This means that the riot (oxidative process) has not worsened. The policemen have not increased because the riots have not gotten out of hand. The prognosis in such cases is not bad, though not always favourable.
2. The second possibility is that uric acid levels have significantly increased. This is a bad prognosis. In the policeman-to-riot model, it means that the policemen have increased in number. It means the rioters are having a field day and the riots are not getting quelled. Because the maternal systems are unable to quell the riots (oxidative reactions), more and more policemen are getting mobilised. This is clinically reflected in increasing levels of uric acid. Failure of intrinsic maternal extracellular reducing systems to neutralise the oxidative reaction means the disease process is still active. In such a situation, the obstetrician needs to intervene or be prepared for an adverse obstetric outcome.
3. The third possibility is that of uric acid levels falling. This means the maternal system has successfully thwarted the disease process. The riots have been quelled, and the policemen have returned home. However, in clinical practice, this hardly ever occurs because the oxidative process is on and so the uric acid levels will not fall until the pregnancy and its effects get over.

LIMITATIONS OF REDUCING SYSTEMS

As is so well-known by now, all actions of ROS are not always pathological. There are many vital functions in the body based on the oxidative process. In the same way, all reducing systems are not necessarily health-promoting. Indeed in the vascular endothelium and ROS are disease-causing, and reducing systems are protective. On the other hand, many reductants also act as oxidizing agents at times. A classic example of this is water-soluble vitamin E analogue Trolox-C. It shows both reducing and oxidative properties in vitro.[56] Such behaviours of some reductants have made clinicians cautious in recommending universal usage of reducing systems.

It is also interesting that any drug system that tries to neutralise health-promoting or health-restoring physiology in the body is met with stiff resistance. The entire system organisation of any living body is to preserve and promote life. If any extraneous, or for that matter, even internal change comes in the way of this orientation of the living system, the latter will make all possible attempts to eliminate it. If total elimination is not possible from the body system, the body will thwart in or blunt it. This explains why large meta-analysis on the efficacy of reducing systems in preventing or treating pre-eclampsia has not shown consistent results. Not all reducing systems are effective. Also, some reducing systems may be partially effective. Some reducing systems may be effective at some times and ineffective at others. Ascorbic acid, for example, has been touted as a supreme reductant meaning; it is effective in combating the oxidative process. However, when ascorbic acid is pharmacologically administered, it is not found to have equally conspicuous results.

A reducing system can be reductant in one setting and an oxidant in another. Interesting results emerged in two bioassays, which highlighted the inconsistent reductant activities of reducing systems. It is now clear that extracellular iron has an important amplifying role in the oxidative process. Extracellular iron amplifies the peroxidation process in the intercellular matrix. In the body serum, ceruloplasmin and apotransferrin play an important role in eliminating these extracellular oxidised lipid particles in which extracellular Fe had an amplification effect. In a study by Cranfield et al., a substantial reduction in the serum-reducing activity of serum ceruloplasmin and apotransferrin was observed in pre-eclampsia, relative to normal pregnancy. This was because in pre-eclampsia, the serum apotransferrin levels were decreased. Thus in pre-eclampsia, the elimination of Fe-amplified lipid peroxides is reduced. On the other hand, a different process occurs concurrently. Reducing system activity (when measured as the ability of the plasma to scavenge water-soluble peroxyl radicals) is increased.[57]

Thus, on one side in pre-eclampsia, the ability of the body to eliminate lipid peroxyl particles decreases, and on the other, in the same body and in the same disease challenge, the scavenging activity of these lipid peroxyl particles is increased. This highlights the consistent inconsistency of the body to respond to an oxidative process. It also shows the inconsistency of body reductants in limiting the oxidant activities. At some level, they limit the pathology, and on other levels, they themselves get limited! This provides vital insights into the question of why inconsistent results are observed in the action of reductants when extraneously administered.

INCONSISTENCY OF REDUCING SYSTEMS

The efficacy of reducing systems can be best summarised as "inconsistent". This is interesting. Simplistically, if the oxidative process should have such a big role in producing pre-eclampsia, reductants must be able to at the least prevent, if not reverse, this condition. But this does not always happen. Also on the experimental platforms, reducing systems produce inconsistent changes. In one trial, vitamins C and E failed to produce a salutary effect on already established pre-eclampsia.[58] Also, vitamin E deficiency is not a characteristic of pre-eclampsia. Vitamin E is one of the most popular antioxidants used by clinicians for many (rational and irrational) indications. Based on the results that have consistently shown the involvement of oxidative stress in the occurrence of pre-eclampsia, the first question asked by average clinicians is: Can vitamin E supplementation solve the problem? The answer from the observations of both in vitro and in vivo studies is a *no*.

As a student of this science, one would, therefore, like to know why the effect of reductants was inconsistent. The answer to this is complex. As has been said in the preceding sections, the oxidative changes are sustaining many physiological mechanisms in the human body. Hence, it seems that

the reducing systems are perceived as agents that can potentially derail these physiological activities. The human body always resists and tries to neutralise any system that will affect its physiology. Universal reductants like vitamin E face resistance to their activity in the body. Therefore, they get neutralised or are inconsistent in their actions. On the other hand, the reducing systems themselves have a changing stance as regards their configuration. By this is meant that there are situations where they behave as reductants as well as oxidative substances. Trolox C, the water-soluble vitamin E analogue is a classic example of this.

THE IDEAL REDUCING SYSTEM

Based on the insights into the aetiopathology of pre-eclampsia and the role of oxidative stress, there is a unique importance of a consistent reducing system. This has eluded science. In nature, it is nearly impossible to find anything ideal. Therefore, it is stated that one should strive for excellence and not perfection. An ideal reducing system, therefore, would be one which reverses the disease process or prevents its occurrence. At the same time, it should not alter, hamper or arrest the ongoing physiology in the body that promotes health. Such an ideal reducing system, which will only and selectively prevent or cure pre-eclampsia is desirable but not available. Until the time that the ideal reducing system is found, a clinician has to either use less than ideal substances. This goes by the principle if you cannot treat the cause, treat the effects.

It also opens up a new concept of desirable and undesirable reducing systems. Undesirable reducing systems would be farthest from the ideal. Desirable reducing systems are those which would be closest to the ideal. The best producer of such desirable reducing systems is the body itself. It is the best organism to judge what can be retained and what can be physiologically detrimental and therefore, be eliminated amongst reducing systems. Exercise, a physiological and health-promoting activity, does this efficiently and classically.

EXERCISE AND PREVENTION OF PRE-ECLAMPSIA

Exercises are a natural phenomenon. There is no extraneous drug sent to the body system to manipulate the body mechanisms. Exercises are a form of "healthy stress" electively produced in the body. It will, therefore, be interesting to study how the body responds to this stress. As exercise is a "physiological stress", the body will respond with distresses that are physiological. If an oxidative process is generated during exercise, the reducing systems generated by exercise would be ideal reducing systems neutralising only the oxidative reaction that produces stress (disease) and not affecting the oxidative reactions that are supporting the physiological processes.

Gavard reported a study on the effects of exercises on some adverse obstetric outcomes, including pre-eclampsia.[59] The purpose of the review was to critically evaluate the scientific literature for the effects of exercise on pregnancy outcomes. Maternal outcomes analysed in this review were gestational diabetes mellitus, pre-eclampsia and weight gain. Foetal outcomes evaluated were birth weight, time of delivery and mode of delivery. Despite methodological pitfalls in the studies published, the evidence suggests a benefit of exercise in pregnancy. Exercise in pregnancy could prevent and limit adverse maternal and foetal morbidities and provide a long-term benefit through the reduction of maternal weight gain during pregnancy and improvement in cardiovascular fitness. Pregnancy emerges as a unique time for behaviour modification.[59] In contrast to this, Meher et al., while reviewing for Cochrane Database, found that there is insufficient evidence for reliable conclusions about the effects of exercise on prevention of pre-eclampsia and its complications.[60]

Nevertheless, when scientists try to estimate the changes in circulating levels of different substances as a result of exercises, they are likely to err on simplicity. The numbers of reducing substances that can be assessed by the human experimental conditions are finite. On the other hand, exercises or such physiological stress are causing changes in infinite and therefore, a massive number of reductants to increase or change. Many of these may still not be known to science.

There are a series of body reducing systems that may not be increased arithmetically in the body. Instead, they simply get activated. This can be similar to the activation of a series of cell linings in immunological responses. Many cells get activated by the mother for eliminating the foreign antigen, the foetus, including platelets. Platelets,

for example, do not increase in arithmetic numbers, but they become functionally more active. Similarly, there are a series of reducing systems in the body that simply get activated without arithmetically increasing in circulation. Consequently, laboratory set-ups can be easily misled into believing that no increase in the particular reducing system occurred, so the said reducing system has no role in preventing or reducing pre-eclampsia through exercises. However, in reality, these may be the most efficient in reducing the effects of oxidative stress.

THE BEAUTY OF LYSOPHOSPHOTIDYL CHOLINE

With the understanding of lipid peroxidation and its effects on endothelial cell activation becoming clear, one more intricate but beautiful phenomenon also gets elucidated. This is the paradoxical phenomenon of healing by the injuring agents. As it is evident, the peroxidised lipid molecules have two critical bearings in the aetiopathology of pre-eclampsia. First is the direct effect on the vascular smooth muscles by tipping the thromboxane-prostacyclin balance. Second is the activation of endothelial cells through sublethal injury. Sublethal injury leads to a release of a myriad of substances, including endothelin. Whereas prostaglandin-thromboxane initiates vasospasm, molecules like endothelin maintain and amplify the process.

The process of injury and disease is ongoing simultaneously. The peroxidised lipid molecules while causing injury concurrently start the healing and neutralising process. It is now known that lysophosphotidyl choline, a component of oxidatively modified LDL, upregulates NOS.[49] This, in simple terms, means it enhances the production of NOS. The NOS increase leads to increased synthesis of NO. An enhanced NO production leads to an increased availability of NO. NO is known to be one of the strongest vasodilators. Thus, the total effect of peroxidised lipid molecules on the vessel wall is vasospasm. But lysophosphotidyl choline generated through the same oxidative process leads to neutralisation of vasospasm and causes vasodilatation. This contradiction is unique. It provides valuable insight into the understanding of the pathophysiology of pre-eclampsia.

This can have therapeutic bearing in clinical practice. The need would be for agents that generate, enhance or amplify the production or action of molecules like lysophosphotidyl choline. If such substances are produced, the process of oxidative stress would not be arrested, but its combative and neutralising systems would be enhanced. This could be the ideal treatment for pre-eclampsia. Such a treatment modality would be close to the ideal reducing system. Such agents would have the capacity to reverse the process of pre-eclampsia. Therefore, their predominant role would not be in the prevention of pre-eclampsia but in reversing and treating them.

Currently, all efforts are confined to use reducing systems to neutralise oxidative stress and its effects. This has given limited results. The other set of management strategies for pre-eclampsia is by preventing its effects because the cause could not be neutralised. Agents like lysophosphotidyl choline hold a promise as the next generation of pharmacological treatment of pre-eclampsia.

REFERENCES

1. Jebbink J, Wolters A, Fernando F, Afink G, van der Post J, Ris-Stalpers C: Molecular genetics of preeclampsia and HELLP syndrome—A review. *Biochem Biophys Acta* 1822(12):1960–1969, 2012. doi:10.1016/j.bbadis.2012.08.004. Epub 2012 Aug 16.
2. Haram K, Mortensen JH, Nagy B: Genetic aspects of preeclampsia and the HELLP syndrome. *J Pregnancy* 2014:910751, 2014. doi:10.1155/2014/910751. Epub 2014 Jun 2.
3. Desai P, Rathod S, Garge V, Mansuri Z: Evaluation of pro-oxidants and antioxidants in preeclampsia. *J Obstet Gynecol India* 53(5):445–448, 2003.
4. Desai P: Reducing systems in preeclampsia. In S. Dasgupta, editor: *Recent Advances in Obstetrics and Gynecology-6*, pp. 79–98, 2003, New Delhi, Jaypee Publishers.
5. Duran M, Schutgens RB, Ketel A, Heymans H, Bertssen MW, Ketting D, Wadman SK: 3-hydroxy-3-methylglutaryl coenzyme A lyase deficiency: Postnatal management following prenatal diagnosis by analysis of maternal urine. *J Pediatr* 95(6):1004–1007, 1979.
6. Neboh E, Emeh J, Aniebue U, Ikekpeazu E, Maduka I, Ezeugwu F: Relationship between lipid and lipoprotein metabolism in trimesters of pregnancy in Nigerian women: Is pregnancy a risk factor. *J Nat Sci Biol Med* 3(1):32–37, 2012.
7. Mouzon SH, Lassance L: Endocrine and metabolic adaptations to pregnancy; impact of obesity. *Horm Mol Biol Clin Investig* 24(1):65–72, 2015. doi:10.1515/hmbci-2015-0042.
8. Newbern D, Freemark M: Placental hormones and the control of maternal metabolism and fetal growth. *Curr Opin Endocrinol Diabetes Obes* 18(6):409–416, 2011.
9. Handwerger S, Freemark M: The roles of placental growth hormone and placental lactogen in the regulation of human fetal growth and development. *J Pediatr Endocrinol Metab* 13(4):343–356, 2000.
10. Mittal P, Hassan S, Espinoza J, Kusanovic J, Edwin S, Gotsch F, Erez O, Than N, Mazaki-Tovi S, Romero R: The effect of gestational age and labor on placental growth hormone in amniotic fluid. *Growth Horm IGF Res* 18(2):174–179, 2008.
11. Woollett LA: Review: Maternal cholesterol in fetal development: Transport of cholesterol from the maternal to the fetal circulation. *Am J Clin Nutr* 82(6):1155–1161, 2005.
12. Hubel C, McLaughlin M, Evans R, Hauth B, Sims C, Roberts J: Fasting serum triglycerides, free fatty acids, and malondialdehyde are increased in preeclampsia, are positively correlated, and decrease within 48 hours postpartum. *Am J Obstet Gynecol* 174(3):975–982, 1996.
13. Lei Q, Lv L, Zhang B, Wen JY, Liu G, Lin X, Niu J: Ante-partum and post-partum markers of metabolic syndrome in preeclampsia. *J Hum Hypertens* 25(1):11–17, 2011.
14. Gosmanov AR, Smiley DD, Peng L, et al.: Vascular effects of intravenous intralipid and dextrose infusions in obese subjects. *Metabolism* 61(10):1370–1376, 2012. doi:10.1016/j.metabol.2012.03.006.
15. Prónai L, Hiramatsu K, Saigusa Y, Nakazawa H: Low superoxide scavenging activity associated with enhanced superoxide generation by monocytes from male hypertriglyceridemia with and without diabetes. *Atherosclerosis* 90(1):39–47, 1991.

16. Heyden S, Heiss G, Manegold C, Tyroler HA, Hames CG, Bartel AG, Cooper G: The combined effect of smoking and coffee drinking on LDL and HDL cholesterol. *Circulation* 60:22–25, 1979. doi:10.1161/01.CIR.60.1.22.

17. Davidson M: Update on CETP inhibition. *J Clin Lipidol* 4(5):394–398, 2010. doi:10.1016/j.jacl.2010.08.003.

18. Czyzewska M, Wolska A, Cwiklińska A, Kortas-Stempak B, Wróblewska M: Disturbances of lipoprotein metabolism in metabolic syndrome. *Postepy Hig Med Dosw* 64:1–10, 2010.

19. Galeano NF, Al-Haideri M, Keyserman F, Rumsey SC, Deckelbaum RJ: Small dense low density lipoprotein has increased affinity for LDL receptor-independent cell surface binding sites: A potential mechanism for increased atherogenicity. *J Lipid Res* 39(6):1263–1273, 1998.

20. Siri-Tarino P, Woods A, Bray G, Krauss R: Reversal of small, dense LDL subclass phenotype by weight loss is associated with impaired fat oxidation. *Obesity* 19(1):61–68, 2011.

21. Austin M, Edwards K: Small, dense low density lipoproteins, the insulin resistance syndrome and noninsulin-dependent diabetes. *Curr Opin Lipidol* 7(3):167–171, 1996.

22. Shia W, Ku T, Tsao Y, Hsia C, Chang Y, Huang C, Chung Y, Hsu S, Liang K, Hsu F: Genetic copy number variants in myocardial infarction patients with hyperlipidemia. *BMC Genomics* 12 Suppl 3:S23, 2011.

23. Kim O, Chung H, Shin M: Higher levels of serum triglyceride and dietary carbohydrate intake are associated with smaller LDL particle size in healthy Korean women. *Nutr Res Pract* 6(2):120–125, 2012.

24. Miranda Guisado M, Vallejo-Vaz A, García Junco P, Jiménez L, García Morillo S, Muñiz Grijalvo O, Alfaro Lara V, Villar Ortiz J, Pamies-Andréu E: Abnormal levels of antioxidant defenses in a large sample of patients with hypertensive disorders of pregnancy. *Hypertens Res* 35(3):274–278, 2012.

25. Genc H, Uzun H, Benian A, Simsek G, Gelisgen R, Madazli R, Güralp O: Evaluation of oxidative stress markers in first trimester for assessment of preeclampsia risk. *Arch Gynecol Obstet* 284(6):1367–1373, 2011.

26. Feng YC, Liao CY, Xia WK, Jiang XZ, Shang F, Yuan GR, Wang JJ: Regulation of three isoforms of SOD gene by environmental stresses in citrus red mite, *Panonychus citri. Exp Appl Acarol* 67(1):49–63, 2015. doi:10.1007/s10493-015-9930-3. Epub 2015 Jun 11.

27. Basu AK, Marnett LJ: Unequivocal demonstration that malondialdehyde is a mutagen. *Carcinogenesis* 4(3):331–333, 1983. doi:10.1093/carcin/4.3.331.

28. Desai P, Patel P, Rathod SP, Mahajan S: Selenium levels and glutathione peroxidase activity in spontaneous inevitable abortion. *J Obstet Gynecol India* 56(4):311–315, 2006.

29. Becker B, Massoudy P, Permanetter B, Raschke P, Zahler S: Possible significance of free oxygen radicals for reperfusion injury. *Z Kardiol* 82(Suppl 5):49–58, 1993.

30. Halliwell B, Gutteridge JM: Oxygen toxicity, oxygen radicals, transition metals and disease. *Biochem J* 219:1–14, 1984.

31. Freeman B, White C, Gutierrez H, Paler-Martínez A, Tarpey M, Rubbo H: Oxygen radical-nitric oxide reactions in vascular diseases. *Adv Pharmacol* 34:45–69, 1995.

32. Urmalia V, Rathod SP: Neurological and Oxidative Stress Assessment: Dissertation submitted to Department of Pharmacy, M.S. University of Baroda.

33. Sahlin L, Wang H, Stjernholm Y, Lundberg M, Ekman G, Holmgren A, Eriksson H: The expression of glutaredoxin is increased in the human cervix in term pregnancy and immediately post-partum, particularly after prostaglandin-induced delivery. *Mol Hum Reprod* 6(12):1147–1153, 2000.

34. Shibata E, Ejima K, Nanri H, Toki N, Koyama C, Ikeda M, Kashimura M: Enhanced protein levels of protein thiol/disulphide oxidoreductases in placentae from pre-eclamptic subjects. *Placenta* 22(6):566–572, 2001.

35. Okatani Y, Wakatsuki A, Shinohara K, Taniguchi K, Fukaya T: Melatonin protects against oxidative mitochondrial damage induced in rat placenta by ischemia and reperfusion. *J Pineal Res* 31(2):173–178, 2001

36. Twina G, Sheiner E, Shahaf G, Salem S, Madar T, Baron J, Wiznitzer A, Mazor M, Holcberg G, Lewis E: Lower circulation levels and activity of alpha-1 antitrypsin in pregnant women with severe preeclampsia. *J Matern Fetal Neonatal Med* 25(12):2667–2670, 2012.

37. Chakraborty D, Rumi MA, Soares MJ: NK cells, hypoxia and trophoblast cell differentiation. *Cell Cycle* 11(13):2427–2430, 2012. doi:10.4161/cc.20542.

38. Maynard SE, Min JY, Merchan J, Lim KH, Li J, Mondal S, Libermann TA et al.: Excess placental soluble fms-like tyrosine kinase 1 (sFlt1) may contribute to endothelial dysfunction, hypertension, and proteinuria in preeclampsia. *J Clin Invest* 111(5):649–658, 2003. doi:10.1172/JCI17189.

39. Luo H, Kimura K, Aoki M, Hirako M: Vascular endothelial growth factor (VEGF) promotes the early development of bovine embryo in the presence of cumulus cells. *J Vet Med Sci* 64(11):967–971, 2002.

40. Donnez J, Smoes P, Gillerot S, Casanas-Roux F, Nisolle M: Vascular endothelial growth factor (VEGF) in endometriosis. *Hum Reprod* 13(6):1686–1690, 1998.

41. Bussen S, Bussen D: Influence of the vascular endothelial growth factor on the development of severe preeclampsia or HELLP syndrome. *Arch Gynecol Obstet* 284(3):551–557, 2011.

42. Chaiworapongsa T, Romero R, Kim Y, Kim G, Kim M, Espinoza J, Bujold E et al.: Plasma soluble vascular endothelial growth factor receptor-1 concentration is elevated prior to the clinical diagnosis of preeclampsia. *J Matern Fetal Neonatal Med* 17(1):3–18, 2005.

43. Akolekar R, de Cruz J, Foidart J, Munaut C, Nicolaides K: Maternal plasma soluble fms-like tyrosine kinase-1 and free vascular endothelial growth factor at 11 to 13 weeks of gestation in preeclampsia. *Prenat Diagn* 30(3):191–197, 2010.

44. Hoffmann P, Saoudi Y, Benharouga M, Graham CH, Schaal JP, Mazouni C, Feige JJ, Alfaidy N: Role of EG-VEGF in human placentation: Physiological and pathological implications. *J Cell Mol Med* 13(8B):2224–2235, 2009.

45. Di Paolo S, Volpe P, Grandaliano G, Stallone G, Schena A, Greco P, Resta L et al.: Increased placental expression of tissue factor is associated with abnormal uterine and umbilical Doppler waveforms in severe preeclampsia with fetal growth restriction. *J Nephrol* 16(5):650–657, 2003.

46. Cho E, Park M, Kim S, Kang G, Choi S, Lee Y, Chang S et al.: Vasorelaxing activity of *Ulmusda vidiana* ethanol extracts in rats: Activation of endothelial nitric oxide synthase. *Korean J Physiol Pharmacol* 15(6):339–344, 2011.

47. Baker P, Krasnow J, Roberts J, Yeo K: Elevated serum levels of vascular endothelial growth factor in patients with preeclampsia. *Obstet Gynecol* 86(5):815–821, 1995.

48. Davidge S, Signorella A, Hubel C, Lykins D, Roberts J: Distinct factors in plasma of preeclamptic women increase endothelial nitric oxide or prostacyclin. *Hypertension* 28(5):758–764, 1996.

49. Hirata K, Miki N, Kuroda Y, Sakoda T, Kawashima S, Yokoyama M: Low concentration of oxidized low-density lipoprotein and lysophosphatidylcholine upregulate constitutive nitric oxide synthase mRNA expression in bovine aortic endothelial cells. *Circ Res* 76(6):958–962, 1995.

50. Rubbo H, Freeman BA: Nitric oxide regulation of lipid oxidation reactions: Formation and analysis of nitrogen-containing oxidized lipid derivatives. *Methods Enzymol* 269:385–394, 1996.

51. Taylor R, Roberts J: Endothelial cell dysfunction: In Lindheimer M, Roberts J, Cunningham F, editors: *Chesley's Hypertensive Disorders of Pregnancy*, Ct. Ed 2, pp. 395–430, Stamford, CT, Appleton & Lange.

52. Sheppard BL, Bonnar J: An ultrastructural study of uteroplacental spiral arteries in hypertensive and normotensive pregnancy and fetal growth retardation. *Br J Obstet Gynecol* 88(7):695–705, 1981.

53. Pierucci F, Piazze Garnica J, Cosmi E, Anceschi M: Oxidability of low density lipoproteins in pregnancy-induced hypertension. *Br J Obstet Gynecol* 103(11):1159–1161, 1996.

54. Munné-Bosch S: The role of alpha-tocopherol in plant stress tolerance. *J Plant Physiol* 162(7):743–748, 2005.

55. Ayala A, Muñoz MF, Argüelles S: Lipid peroxidation: Production, metabolism, and signaling mechanisms of malondialdehyde and 4-hydroxy-2-nonenal. *Oxid Med Cell Longev* 2014, 2014. doi:10.1155/2014/360438.

56. Albertini R, Abuja PM: Prooxidant and antioxidant properties of Trolox C, analogue of vitamin E, in oxidation of low-density lipoprotein. *Free Radic Res* 30(3):181–188, 1999.

57. Cranfield L, Gollan J, White A, Dormandy T: Serum antioxidant activity in normal and abnormal subjects. *Ann Clin Biochem* 16(6):299–306, 1979.

58. Polyzos NP, Tzioras S, Mauri D, Papanikolaou EG: Combined vitamin C and E supplementation for preeclampsia: No significant effect but significant heterogeneity? *Hypertens Pregnancy* 31(3):375–376, 2012. doi:10.3109/10641955.2010.507852. Epub 2010 Sep 7.

59. Gavard JA, Artal R: Effect of exercise on pregnancy outcome. *Clin Obstet Gynecol* 51(2):467–480, 2008.

60. Meher S, Duley L: Exercise or other physical activity for preventing pre-eclampsia and its complications. *Cochrane Database Syst Rev* 2006(2):CD005942, 2006 Apr 19. doi:10.1002/14651858.CD005942.

5

Metabolic syndrome and pre-eclampsia

WHAT IS METABOLIC SYNDROME?

The clusters of conditions that comprise MS increase the risk of heart attack, diabetes, and even stroke. MS has many names. It is called "syndrome X", "insulin resistance syndrome", "Reaven syndrome", and "the deadly quartet". Currently, it is estimated that there are 1 million new cases of MS diagnosed every year in India. In a cross-sectional study conducted in three districts in Kerala, India, covering more than 5,000 participants, 1 of 4 individuals had ATP III MS (24%). The prevalence estimates were even higher when using the International Diabetes Federation (IDF) and Harmonization definitions (29% and 33%, respectively).[1]

METABOLIC SYNDROME AND HYPERTENSION

As the focus of this topic is MS in relation to pre-eclampsia, it was thought to be prudent to first examine the association between MS and hypertension. Insulin resistance, obesity, atherogenic dyslipidaemia and hypertension, which comprise MS are interrelated and share underlying mediators, mechanisms and pathways. Though there is no agreement on the exact aetiology of MS, insulin resistance probably has a key role in its causation. In 1988, Gerald Reaven gave the Banting Lecture at the American Diabetes Association national meeting and introduced the concept of what he called "Syndrome X", which later became the accepted term, MS. Reaven strongly hinted at the role insulin resistance played in causing MS. In 1991, an article titled "Hyperinsulinemia: The key feature of a cardiovascular and MS", reflected Reaven's viewpoint better.[2] Support for the role of hyperinsulinemia in causing MS came in 1992 when it was reported from an 8 years' prospective data of 2217 subjects that fasting hyperinsulinemia preceded the development of other aspects of the syndrome, including hypertension, hypertriglyceridemia and depressed HDL-C, as well as the development of type II diabetes.[3] Reaven suggested in his lecture some mechanisms to explain how insulin resistance and hyperinsulinemia might cause the other aspects of MS. He pointed out that hypertension was associated with elevated levels of plasma catecholamines and suggested an enhanced sympathetic nervous system activity as a contributing mechanism. It was suggested in a review that hyperinsulinemia was associated with hypertension and could be the result of several mechanisms, including an overactive sympathetic nervous system, sodium retention, altered membrane ion transport and proliferation of vascular smooth muscle cells.[4]

In an attempt to clear up some of the controversies and unify the clinical definitions of MS, a meeting was convened with representatives from the IDF Task Force on Epidemiology and Prevention; National Heart, Lung and Blood Institute (NHLBI); American Heart Association (AHA); World Heart Federation; International Atherosclerosis Society; and International Association for the Study of

Table 5.1 Established criteria proposed for clinical diagnosis of metabolic syndrome

Clinical measure	WHO (1998)	IDF (2005)	Joint IDR/NHLBI/AHA
Insulin resistance	IGT, IFT, T2DM, or lowered insulin sensitivity[a] Plus any two of the following	None	None But any three of the following five features
Body metric	Men: waist-to-hip ratio >0.90 Women: waist-to-hip ratio >0.85 and/or BMI >30 kg/m²	Increased WC (population specific) plus any two of the following	Population- and country-specific definitions
Lipid	TG 150 mg/dL and/or HDL-C <35 mg/dL in men or <39 mg/dL in women	TG >150 mg/dL or on TG Rx HDL-C <40 mg/dL in men or <50 mg/dL in women or on HDL-C Rx	≥150 mg/dL (1.7 mmol/L) <40 mg/dL (1.0 mmol/L) in males; <50 mg/dL (1.3 mmol/L) in females
Blood pressure	≥140/90 mmHg	≥130 mmHg systolic or 85 mmHg diastolic or on hypertension Rx	Systolic ≥130 and/or diastolic ≥85 mmHg
Glucose	IGT, IFG or T2DM	≥100 mg/dL (includes diabetes)	≥100 mg/dL
Other	Microalbuminuria		

Source: Alberti, K.G. et al., Circulation, 120: 1640–1645, 2009.
Note: Metabolic syndrome criteria as defined by WHO, IDF, and the joint IDR/NHLBI/AHA are compared.
Abbreviations: AHA, American Heart Association; BMI, body mass index; HDL-C, high-density lipoprotein-cholesterol; IDF, International Diabetes Federation Task Force on Epidemiology and Prevention; IDR, Integrated Data Repository; IFG, impaired fasting glucose; IGT, impaired glucose tolerance; NHLBI, National Heart, Lung and Blood Institute; Rx, prescription; T2DM indicates type 2 diabetes mellitus; TG, triglycerides; WC, waist circumferences.
[a] Insulin sensitivity measured under hyperinsulinemic euglycemic conditions, glucose uptake below lowest quartile for background population under investigation.

Obesity. In 2009, a "joint interim statement" was published in Circulation, attempting to establish criteria to identify patients with MS as shown in Table 5.1.[5]

MS may also amplify hypertension-related cardiac and renal changes, over and above the potential contribution of every single component of this syndrome.[6] Angiotensin disturbance supposedly plays an important role in causing hypertension in individuals who are obese with MS. Angiotensin II, a potent vasoconstrictor, may trigger the increased incidence of obesity-associated hypertension. This notion is supported in rodent models where hypertension and increased fat mass were observed in animals with an adipose selective overexpression of angiotensin II.[7]

METABOLIC CHANGES IN NORMAL PREGNANCY

Pregnancy has profound changes in all physiological processes in pregnancy. Expectedly, therefore, metabolic changes are also likely to be significant. Foetal demands and a woman's own changes, like that in the breasts, are big contributors to these changes. Also, reserves must be generated to meet the additional needs put on a woman's body during pregnancy, childbirth and the postpartum period.

Basal metabolic rate

The basal metabolic rate (BMR) commences its rise in the late first trimester and can rise up to double the non-pregnant rate by the time a woman approaches delivery. Interestingly, this rise is in proportion to the increase in the size of the foetus. This rise can be falsely attributed to be indicative of an increase in thyroid activity. Gestational diabetes mellitus (GDM) is the most common metabolic disorder during pregnancy. Both BMR and GDM have been linked with gestational weight gain, a fact suggesting a possible association between them.[8] Conditions like adolescent pregnancies post an additional burden on the body of the mother because the young mother is also still developing. As a result, BMR changes can be more pronounced in this group of pregnant mothers.

Proteins and amino acids

During pregnancy, nitrogen which is obtained from the metabolism of consumed protein is wanted for growth of the foetus, the placenta, the uterus and mother's breasts and other tissues. A substantial amount of nitrogen also is essential for the rise in the mother's red cell volume and plasma. Protein deposition in maternal and foetal tissues increases throughout pregnancy, with most occurring during the third trimester. Dietary protein intake recommendations are based on factorial estimates because the traditional method of determining protein requirements, nitrogen balance, is invasive and undesirable during pregnancy. The current estimated average requirement and recommended daily allowance (RDA) recommendations is of 0.88–1.1 g/kg for all stages of pregnancy. The single recommendation does not take into account the changing needs during different stages of pregnancy. Recently, this was recalibrated to an average of 1.2 and 1.52 $g/kg^{(-1)}/d^{(-1)}$ during early (~16 weeks) and late (~36 weeks) stages of pregnancy, respectively.[9]

Carbohydrates

In early pregnancy, basal glucose and insulin concentrations do not differ significantly from non-gravid values.[10] Basal hepatic glucose production does not differ at 12–14 weeks of gestation. By the third trimester, however, basal glucose concentrations are 10–15 mg/dL (0.56–0.83 mmol/L) lower and insulin is almost twice the concentration of non-gravid women. Post-prandial glucose

concentrations are significantly elevated, and the glucose peak is prolonged.[11] Basal endogenous hepatic glucose production increases by 16%–30% to meet the increasing needs of the placenta and foetus.[10,12,13] Glucose production increases with maternal body weight, such that glucose production per kilogram body weight does not change throughout pregnancy.[13] Endogenous glucose production remains sensitive to increased insulin concentration throughout gestation (90% suppression), in contrast with the progressive decrease in peripheral insulin sensitivity.[14]

Commensurate with the increased rate of glucose appearance, studies have shown an increased contribution of carbohydrate to oxidative metabolism in late pregnancy.[14] Measured by respiration calorimetry, the 24-h respiratory quotient (RQ) is significantly higher in late pregnancy than postpartum, such that carbohydrate oxidation as a percentage of non-protein energy expenditure decreases from 66% to 58% from late pregnancy to 6 months postpartum.[15] Absolute rates of carbohydrate oxidation are significantly higher in pregnancy (282 g/d) than postpartum (210 g/d). The RQs during measurements of BMR and sleeping metabolic rate are also higher during pregnancy.[14]

Lipids

The changes in hepatic and adipose metabolism alter circulating concentrations of triacylglycerols, fatty acids, cholesterol and phospholipids.[16] After an initial decrease in the first 8 weeks of pregnancy, there is a steady increase in triacylglycerols, fatty acids, cholesterol, lipoproteins and phospholipids. The higher concentration of oestrogen and insulin resistance are thought to be responsible for the hypertriglyceridemia of pregnancy.[14] Changes in total cholesterol concentration reflect changes in the various lipoprotein fractions. HDL cholesterol increased by 12 weeks of gestation in response to oestrogen and remains elevated throughout pregnancy.[17] Total and low-density lipoprotein-cholesterol (LDL-C) concentrations decrease initially but then increase in the second and third trimesters. Very-low-density lipoprotein (VLDL) and triacylglycerols decrease in the first 8 weeks of gestation and then continuously increase until term.[14]

DIAGNOSIS OF METABOLIC SYNDROME

According to guidelines from the NHLBI and the AHA, MS is diagnosed when a patient has at least three of the following five conditions:

1. Fasting glucose ≥100 mg/dL (or receiving drug therapy for hyperglycaemia)
2. Blood pressure ≥130/85 mmHg (or receiving drug therapy for hypertension)
3. Triglycerides ≥150 mg/dL (or receiving drug therapy for hypertriglyceridemia)
4. HDL-C <40 mg/dL in men or <50 mg/dL in women (or receiving drug therapy for reduced HDL-C)
5. Waist circumference ≥102 cm (40 in) in men or ≥88 cm (35 in) in women; if Asian American, ≥90 cm (35 in) in men or ≥80 cm (32 in) in women.

METABOLIC SYNDROME AND PRE-ECLAMPSIA

With the association between MS and hypertension now well established, one would like to know if that association can be extended to pre-eclampsia. In a prospective study carried out in Iran, it was found that in women with the MS during pregnancy, the risk for pre-eclampsia in the second half of pregnancy was higher than in the general population.[18] In a Chinese study, 62 women with a history of severe pre-eclampsia 1 to 3 years after an indexed pregnancy were studied. It was found that an unfavourable metabolic constitution in women may lead to MS, pre-eclampsia and long-term cardiovascular disease. The authors recommend that in women with severe pre-eclampsia, therapeutic interventions should include weight control shortly after pregnancy, especially among women who were previously overweight.[19]

The Iranian study indirectly indicates that late-onset pre-eclampsia is more likely in subjects with MS.[18] However, looking at the aetiopathology of both conditions, it seems the early-onset pre-eclampsia seems to be more likely. This is indeed found in another study with a larger number of subjects and better study design. It was found that the prevalence of the MS postpartum is twice as high in women with a history of early-onset (delivery before 34 weeks) compared to late-onset vascular-complicated pregnancy (delivery at or beyond 34 weeks).[20] The level of evidence was II. Interestingly, it has been suggested that it is important for long-term follow-up assessment for cardiovascular risk factors in subjects with pre-eclampsia.[21]

Results from these different studies suggest that subjects with clinical manifestation of MS have a higher chance of developing pre-eclampsia remote from term and even other obstetric vasculopathies. Not only does it stop with pregnancy, but after pregnancy, subjects with obstetric vasculopathies can develop MS at a later date. So, like women who deliver large-for-gestational-age babies should be kept under observation for development of diabetes, so should women with pre-eclampsia remote from term and other vasculopathies be kept under observation for development of MS. One is inclined to think that lifestyle changes that prevent excessive weight gain should be recommended to these women if a history of polycystic ovary syndrome (PCOS), diabetes mellitus or obesity runs in their families. Also in subjects with MS who conceive, preventive measures like low-dose aspirin and measures of early detection like uterine artery colour Doppler during the first trimester scan can be of great help.

REFERENCES

1. Harikrishnan S, Sarma S, Sanjay G, Jeemon P, Krishnan M N, Venugopal K, Mohanan P P et al.: Prevalence of metabolic syndrome and its risk factors in Kerala, South India: Analysis of a community based cross-sectional study. *PLoS One* 13(3):e0192372, 2018. doi:10.1371/journal.pone.0192372.
2. Ferrannini E, Haffner SM, Mitchell BD, Stern MP: Hyperinsulinaemia: The key feature of a cardiovascular and metabolic syndrome. *Diabetologia* 34(6):416–422, 1991.
3. Haffner SM, Valdez RA, Hazuda HP, Mitchell BD, Morales PA, Stern MP: Prospective analysis of the insulin-resistance syndrome (syndrome X). *Diabetes* 41(6):715–722, 1992.
4. Baron AD: Hemodynamic actions of insulin. *Am J Physiol* 267(2 Pt 1):E187–E202, 1994.
5. Alberti KG, Eckel RH, Grundy SM, Zimmet PZ, Cleeman JI, Donato KA, Fruchart JC, James WP, Loria CM, Smith SC Jr: International Diabetes Federation Task Force

on Epidemiology and Prevention, National Heart, Lung, and Blood Institute, American Heart Association, World Heart Federation, International Atherosclerosis Society, International Association for the Study of Obesity. *Circulation* 120(16).1640–1645, 2009.

6. Mulè G, Nardi E, Cottone S, Cusimano P, Volpe V, Piazza G, Mongiovì R et al.: Influence of metabolic syndrome on hypertension-related target organ damage. *J Intern Med* 257(6):503–513, 2005.

7. Massiéra F, Bloch-Faure M, Ceiler D, Murakami K, Fukamizu A, Gasc JM, Quignard-Boulange A et al.: Adipose angiotensinogen is involved in adipose tissue growth and blood pressure regulation. *FASEB J* 15(14):2727–2729, 2001.

8. Taousani E, Savvaki D, Tsirou E, Poulakos P, Mintziori G, Zafrakas M, Vavilis D, Goulis DG: Regulation of basal metabolic rate in uncomplicated pregnancy and in gestational diabetes mellitus. *Hormones (Athens)* 16(3):235–250, 2017. doi:10.14310/horm.2002.1743.

9. Elango R, Ball RO: Protein and amino acid requirements during pregnancy. *Adv Nutr* 7(4):839S–844S, 2016. doi:10.3945/an.115.011817.

10. Catalano PM, Tyzbir ED, Wolfe RR, Roman NM, Amini SB, Sims EAH: Longitudinal changes in basal hepatic glucose production and suppression during insulin infusion in normal pregnant women. *Am J Obstet Gynecol* 167:913–919, 1992.

11. Cousins L, Rigg L, Hollingsworth D: The 24-hour excursion and diurnal rhythm of glucose, insulin, and C-peptide in normal pregnancy. *Am J Obstet Gynecol* 136:483–488, 1980.

12. Kalhan SC, D'Angelo LJ, Savin SM, Adam PAJ: Glucose production in pregnant women at term gestation: Sources of glucose for human fetus. *J Clin Invest* 63:388–394, 1979.

13. Assel B, Rossi K, Kalhan S: Glucose metabolism during fasting through human pregnancy: Comparison of tracer method with respiratory calorimetry. *Am J Physiol* 265:E351–E356, 1993.

14. Butte NF: Carbohydrate and lipid metabolism in pregnancy: Normal compared with gestational diabetes mellitus. *Am J Clin Nutr* 71(5 Suppl):1256S–1261S, 2000. doi: 10.1093/ajcn/71.5.1256s.

15. Butte NF, Hopkinson JM, Mehta N, Moon JK, Smith EO: Adjustments in energy expenditure and substrate utilization during late pregnancy and lactation. *Am J Clin Nutr* 69:299–307, 1999.

16. Lesser KB, Carpenter MW: Metabolic changes associated with normal pregnancy and pregnancy complicated by diabetes mellitus. *Semin Perinatol* 18:399–406, 1994.

17. Halstead AC, Lockitch G, Vallance H, Wadsworth L, Wittmann B: *Handbook of Diagnostic Biochemistry and Hematology in Normal Pregnancy*, 1993, Boca Raton, FL, CRC Press, pp. 3–235.

18. Kianpour M, Norozi S, Bahadoran P, Azadbakht L: The relationship between metabolic syndrome criteria and pre-eclampsia in primigravida women. *Iran J Nurs Midwifery Res* 20(2):263–268, 2015.

19. Lu J, Zhao Y-y, Qiao J, Zhang H-J, Ge Lin, Wei Y: A follow-up study of women with a history of severe preeclampsia: Relationship between metabolic syndrome and pre-eclampsia. *Chin Med J* 124(5):775–779, 2011.

20. Stekkinger E, Zandstra M, Peeters LL, Spaanderman ME: Early-onset preeclampsia and the prevalence of postpartum metabolic syndrome. *Obstet Gynecol* 114(5):1076–1084, 2009. doi:10.1097/AOG.0b013e3181b7b242.

21. Forest JC, Girouard J, Massé J, Moutquin JM, Kharfi A, Ness RB, Roberts JM, Giguère Y: Early occurrence of metabolic syndrome after hypertension in pregnancy. *Obstet Gynecol* 105(6):1373–1380, 2005.

6

The genetics of pre-eclampsia

BASIS FOR REVIEWING THE ROLE OF GENETICS IN PRE-ECLAMPSIA

For quite some time now, scientists have tried to find out if there are some aspects of genetics involved in the process of pre-eclampsia. Based on an observational study, Leon Chesley[1] suggested that pre-eclampsia had some strange tendency to run into families. Still, efforts to find a single and specific gene responsible for pre-eclampsia or other vasculopathies remains fruitless. But some recent studies may be on the threshold of changing the belief that pre-eclampsia is not a disease of polygenic origin.

Over the past decade, genome-wide association studies have allowed for significant advances in the understanding of the genetic basis of many common diseases. Genome-wide association studies are based on the idea that the genetic basis of many common diseases is complex and polygenic with many variants, each with modest effects that contribute to disease risk. Using this approach in pre-eclampsia, a large genome-wide association study recently identified and replicated the first robust foetal genomic region associated with excess risk.[2] In this study, a screen of >7 million genetic variants in 2,658 offspring from women with pre-eclampsia and 308,292 population controls identified a single association signal close to the Fms-like tyrosine kinase 1 gene, on chromosome 13. Fms-like tyrosine kinase 1 (sFlt-1) encodes soluble Fms-like tyrosine kinase 1. It is a splice variant of the vascular endothelial growth factor receptor that exerts antiangiogenic activity by inhibiting signalling of proangiogenic factors. Thus, what began as a chemical parameter to predict pre-eclampsia is likely to reveal the genetic basis of this disease in the time to follow.

It is now believed that one or more relatively common alleles act as "major genes", conferring susceptibility to pre-eclampsia. They act as susceptibility loci. They lower a women's threshold for developing pre-eclampsia.[2] It is likely that the chromosome that bears this allele could be located on chromosome 13.[3]

One interesting question arises from this: Is the emerging genetic picture applicable to all types of pre-eclampsia? The basis of this question is the fact that at least two types of pre-eclampsia have now been identified: The early-onset pre-eclampsia (appearing clinically at or before 34 weeks of pregnancy) and late-onset pre-eclampsia (appearing after 34 weeks of pregnancy). Hints of the genetic basis of late-onset pre-eclampsia have been in circulation for quite some time, and studies may be able to explain this type of pre-eclampsia. However, the bigger challenge for clinicians is pre-eclampsia remote from term. This type of pre-eclampsia has been thought to have a basis at the foetomaternal interface.

In such an emerging picture, it would be interesting to examine the genetic control of the activities at the foetomaternal interface and maternal vasculature response to the same. This may likely be under some genetic control. These genes may be maternal or foetal. The process of generation of ROS, denaturation of lipid molecules, activation of endothelium and generation of vasospasm seem to have a genetic basis. Yet the major point that needs to be understood is the question as to whether the genetic basis causes the entire process or only one of the initiating events. It is

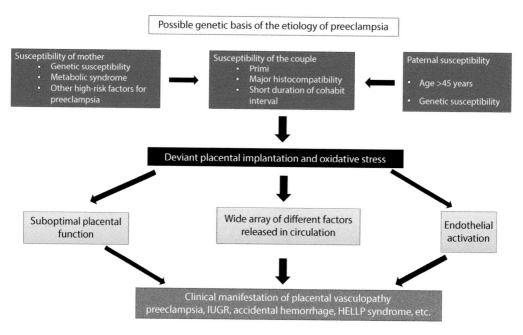

Figure 6.1 Possible genetic basis of the aetiology of pre-eclampsia.

possible that once the key event is initiated, the entire process may be self-maintained through its cyclic and interdependent character. The possible genetic mechanism in causation of pre-eclampsia is shown in Figure 6.1.

CHALLENGES TO THE GENETIC STUDIES IN PRE-ECLAMPSIA

There are at least two types of pre-eclampsia now acknowledged. In this, the early-onset pre-eclampsia is accepted to be mainly a placental problem, with widespread gross and molecular pathologies causing the release of pro-inflammatory and anti-angiogenic factors into the maternal circulation. By contrast, in late-onset pre-eclampsia, the placenta is often indistinguishable from normotensive controls, and evidence of malperfusion is minimal. Instead, it is thought that in these cases, the individuals carry a genetic predisposition to cardiovascular disease, causing them to be vulnerable to even lower levels of factors released from a comparatively normal placenta.

There are many phenotypes of pre-eclampsia like early-onset pre-eclampsia, proteinuric hypertension, haemolysis, elevated liver enzymes, low platelet count, known as the (HELLP) syndrome,

gestational hypertension or pre-eclamptic hypertension superimposed on an under running chronic hypertension. Clear differences have been shown in maternal and foetal characteristics between women who develop preterm pre-eclampsia and those who develop pre-eclampsia at term. Such data support the hypothesis that multiple pre-eclamptic phenotypes exist.[4] Although one subject may have one set of phenotypes, another subject may just have one or most of these features missing. This proves a challenge for the geneticist.

This would become clear by examining an example. Trisomy-21, or mongolism as it is popularly known, can be one such example. The phenotypes of T21 are consistent and regular. The facial features and mental challenges found in the subjects with T21 are found in all its subjects albeit with different intensity. Therefore, it becomes easy for a geneticist to associate the T21 genotype with the phenotype of mongolism. This consistency is completely lacking in pre-eclampsia. Hypertension, which is most consistent and supposed to be most critical, is also inconsistent in its manifestation.

One more challenge for the geneticist in assigning phenotypes to a genetic basis of pre-eclampsia is the fact that all of these are occurring with pregnancy. Pregnancy is a sex-limited trait. What role do the males, therefore, have in this condition is also a matter not yet fully understood.

MAMMALIAN STUDIES

Many interesting studies based on records of mothers, daughters, sisters and even granddaughters of indexed subjects who had pre-eclampsia were undertaken at different instances of time. The principle results of these studies were:

- *Humphries:* Pre-eclampsia occurred in 28% of daughters of mothers who had pre-eclampsia. This incidence was 13% in controls.[5]
- *Chesley:* Rate of pre-eclampsia was higher in mothers, sisters, daughters and granddaughters of subjects who had pre-eclampsia.[1]
- *Aberdeen:* It was found that sisters of women with pre-eclampsia had a 2.1- to 3.4-fold increase in the rate of pre-eclampsia. Mothers of subjects who had pre-eclampsia showed four times higher incidence of the condition compared with mothers of women controls without pre-eclampsia.[6]
- *Procopciuc:* In pre-eclampsia, both maternal and newborn genetic variations implicated in blood pressure regulation are important.[10]

In the absence of any identifiable gene and a set genotype, these studies provide some important leads on the hereditary behaviour of pre-eclampsia. These studies may open a window to the chromosomal basis of these conditions. It becomes obvious from these studies that there is some familial link in pre-eclampsia. This link does not seem to be based on food, living styles or any such confounding variable. The only link that binds these subjects is genes. Also, the fact that these subjects who showed a higher incidence of pre-eclampsia were essentially blood relatives and not related through marriage eliminates the extraneous factors on one hand and reasserts the possible genetic basis on the other.

APPLICATION OF GENETIC MODELS

As has been described in the previous sections, no set pattern of inheritance appears in pre-eclampsia in these studies of the families. Expectedly, therefore, all sorts of inheritance patterns have been suggested. There are some who have suggested a recessive pattern of inheritance. There are others who have also suggested a polygenic origin. Lack of consistency in these results confirms that though there is some genetic factor that plays a role in the inheritance of pre-eclampsia, this role is at best amorphous. However, pre-eclampsia being an autosomal dominant condition is ruled out.

To date, numerous genetic studies, using both the candidate gene and genome-wide approach, have been undertaken to identify the genetic basis of pre-eclampsia, if any. Such studies have identified some promising candidate genes such as STOX1 and ACVR2A. Nevertheless, researchers face ongoing challenges of replicating these genetic associations in different populations and performing the functional validation of identified genetic variants to determine their causality in the disorder.[7]

EXAMINING ASSOCIATIONS

In some strange ways in clinical practice, one finds some apparent association of pre-eclampsia with some genetic conditions. This includes conditions like Beckwith-Wiedemann syndrome and trisomy 13. But these have at best remained associations not maturing to any cause-and-effect relationships.

FOETAL CONTRIBUTIONS: ANY?

The foetomaternal interface seems to have a big role to play in the aetiopathology of pre-eclampsia. It is therefore worthwhile examining the role of foetal genetic contribution in this condition. For this, one has to assess the role of the father. This is because the genetic contribution of the mother in the foetus is similar to her. Therefore, the expression in the foetus would also be similar to the mother. The difference in foetal genetic makeup is from the father.

On pure clinical observational classic study, one is made aware of a gentleman in Utah. It was reported that he lost two of his wives to eclampsia. His third wife also developed severe pre-eclampsia.[8] Another study concluded that a shorter duration of exposure to sperm was more common in women with pre-eclampsia compared with controls.[9]

Arngrimsson had some interesting observations.[10] This study hinted at the possibility of daughters'-in-law of women with pre-eclampsia having a small but distinct chance of developing pre-eclampsia. The daughter-in-law is currently pregnant with a foetus that has genetic contributions from four sources:

1. Her own father,
2. Her own mother,
3. Her husband's father and
4. Her husband's mother.

The father-in-law has indeed a small but distinct genetic contribution in building the foetus being sired by the daughter-in-law of the women who had pre-eclampsia. When Arngrimsson et al. found that there is some association between the history of pre-eclampsia in subjects and their daughters-in-law developing this condition, the association was weak.[10] It means that the subjects did develop pre-eclampsia but did not follow any set genetic model of inheritance. This weakness in association could be attributable to the weakening of paternal genetic material in the foetus sired by the daughter-in-law to one-fourth. Even if the association is amorphous, if Arngrimsson et al. could find some association with pre-eclampsia, in itself these findings are important and noteworthy.

Another abnormal pregnancy condition is a molar pregnancy. These pregnancies may have some leads in regard to the genetic basis of pre-eclampsia. For decades together, scientists and clinicians have found that subjects with vesicular mole have a higher chance of developing pre-eclampsia. This higher chance strongly hints at a paternal contribution. As is well-known, a molar pregnancy has two sets of chromosomes – both paternal. The maternal chromosomes are absent. This absence of maternal chromosomal contribution is because the ovum fertilised in molar pregnancy is a "ghost ovum". It lacks the chromosomal contribution from the mother. In the absence of maternal chromosomal contribution, women develop pre-eclampsia with a much higher and furious intensity. It seems that the father through his chromosomal component in the foetus has a small but important contribution to make in the aetiopathology of pre-eclampsia.

Clinical conditions like recurrent spontaneous miscarriages due to Factor V Leiden mutation and renal conditions resulting from angiotensinogen genetic variations have a higher chance of developing pre-eclampsia. They have a distinct genetic basis.[11] It, therefore, seems possible that there exists some association between pre-eclampsia and genes.

IMMUNOLOGY AND GENETICS

Immunology has been accepted to play a big role in the occurrence of pre-eclampsia. Pre-eclampsia is an obstetric vasculopathy and so are recurrent miscarriages of missed abortion type occurring late in the first trimester and in the second trimester. There can be some common genetic basis for both these conditions. If found in one, there can be a genetic basis in the other.

The foetus is now accepted as an allograft that has a tendency to get rejected by the mother. This is because of the distinctly different antigenicity of the mother and the foetus. There seems to be a constant struggle between the survival efforts of the foetus and the destructive effects of the mother. In preventing and protecting the foetus from rejection and destruction, the trophoblasts play an important role. It has been found that if the foetus and the mother share histocompatibility antigens, there is a distinct chance of rejection. However, the interesting fact is that the sharing of antigens, major histocompatibility antigens (MHC Class 1) or minor histocompatibility antigens (MHC Class 2) is strongly genetic based. One Tunisian study investigated the possible association of natural killer group (NKG) receptors gene polymorphisms and MHC class I chain-related protein A (MICA) gene polymorphism with recurrent miscarriage (RM). It reported that the NKG2D gene polymorphisms may influence the success of pregnancy in Tunisian women.[12]

One interesting study will not be out of place to quote here in this regard. Data from Danish women (1996–2002) with single live-birth pregnancies complicated by severe pre-eclampsia or eclampsia were compared to women with term pregnancies uncomplicated by hypertension. HLA A, B and DR types were resolved at the intermediate-level typing (antigen). The odds ratios of pre-eclampsia or eclampsia in mothers sharing both HLA antigens with their infants were 1.19 for HLA A, 0.91 for HLA B and 1.05 for HLA DR antigens. No specific HLA antigens in either mother or infant appeared important, except possibly DR01 in mothers (protective). Thus, it was concluded that this is not the basis for the mother developing pre-eclampsia or eclampsia.[13]

EPIGENETICS AND PRE-ECLAMPSIA

Based on a mouse model, some workers have indicated that there may be a role of epigenetics in pre-eclampsia. In simple words, epigenetics is the study of changes in organisms caused by modification of gene expression rather than alteration of the genetic code itself. It is currently believed that pre-eclampsia results from epigenetic expression rather than some alteration in genetic codes. Insights have been gained from the analysis of mouse models into the epigenetic mechanisms that are required for the early establishment of the trophoblast line and the development of specialised cell types of the placenta. These insights suggest that the causes and consequences of a variety of placental pathologies are related to epigenetic processes. Furthermore, the epigenetic landscape that regulates trophoblast cells seems to be particularly vulnerable to alterations during the development. These crucial insights form the basis for suggesting some epigenetic basis for pre-eclampsia and extended to other vasculopathies. Initial results suggest that the causes and consequences of a variety of placental pathologies are related to epigenetic pathways.[14]

Pregnancy is known to induce rapid, progressive and substantial changes to the cardiovascular system, ultimately facilitating successful pregnancy outcomes. Women who develop hypertensive disorders during pregnancy are considered to have "failed" the cardiovascular stress test of pregnancy. Offspring born to mothers with pre-eclampsia exhibit an elevated risk of cardiovascular disease, stroke and mental disorders during adulthood. This suggests that pre-eclampsia not only exposes the mother and the foetus to complications during pregnancy but also programs chronic diseases during adulthood in the offspring. Although it is not clear whether immunological alterations occur early during pregnancy, studies have proposed that dysregulated systemic and placental immunity contributes to impaired angiogenesis and the onset of pre-eclampsia. Recently, strong evidence have suggested a potential link among epigenetics, micro RNAs (miRNAs), and pregnancy complications.[15]

In times to follow, it can explain many hidden enigmas of pre-eclampsia.

REFERENCES

1. Chesley L: Hypertension in pregnancy; Definitions, familial factor, and remote prognosis. *Kidney Int* 18(2):234–240, 1980.
2. Ward K, Lindheimer M, Roberts J: Endothelial cell dysfunction. In Lindheimer M, Roberts J, Cunningham F, editors: *Chesley's Hypertensive Disorders of Pregnancy*, 2nd ed., pp. 431–452, 1999, Stamford, CT, Appleton & Lange.
3. Gray KJ, Saxena R, Karumanchi SA: Genetic predisposition to preeclampsia is conferred by fetal DNA variants near FLT1, a gene involved in the regulation of angiogenesis. *Am J Obstet Gynecol* 218(2):211–218, 2018. doi:10.1016/j.ajog.2017.11.562.
4. Phillips JK, Janowiak M, Badger GJ, Bernstein IM: Evidence for distinct preterm and term phenotypes of preeclampsia. *J Matern Fetal Neonatal Med* 23(7):622–626, 2010. doi:10.3109/14767050903258746.
5. Humphries J: Occurrence of hypertensive toxemia of pregnancy. *Obstet Gynecol* 107: 271–277, 1960.
6. Adams EM, Finlayson A: Familial aspects of pre-eclampsia and hypertension in pregnancy. *Lancet* 2(7217):1375–1378, 1961. doi:10.1016/s0140-6736(61)91197-7.
7. Yong HEJ, Murthi P, Brennecke SP, Moses EK: Genetic approaches in preeclampsia. *Methods Mol Biol* 1710:53–72, 2018. doi: 10.1007/978-1-4939-7498-6_5.
8. Astin M, Scott J, Worley R: 1981. Preeclampsia: Eclampsia: The fatal father factor. *Lancet* 2(8245):533, 1981.
9. Sadat Z, Abedzadeh Kalahroudi M, Saberi F: The effect of short duration sperm exposure on development of preeclampsia in primigravid women. *Iran Red Crescent Med J* 14(1):20–24, 2012.
10. Arngrimsson R, Bjornson S, Geirsson R et al.: Genetic and familial predisposition to eclampsia and preeclampsia in a defined population. *Br J Obstet Gynecol* 97, 762–769, 1990.
11. von Tempelhoff GF, Heilmann L, Spanuth E, Kunzmann E, Hommel G: Incidence of the factor V Leiden-mutation, coagulation

inhibitor deficiency, and elevated antiphospholipid-antibodies in patients with pre-eclampsia or HELLP-syndrome: Haemolysis, elevated liver-enzymes, low platelets. *Thromb Res* 100(4):363–365, 2000.

12. Hizem S, Mtiraoui N, Massaoudi S, Fortier C, Boukouaci W, Kahina A, Charron D, Mahjoub T, Tamouza R: Polymorphisms in genes coding for the NK-cell receptor NKG2D and its ligand MICA in recurrent miscarriage. *Am J Reprod Immunol* 72(6):577–585, 2014. doi:10.1111/aji.12314.

13. Biggar R, Poulsen G, Ng J, Melbye M, Boyd H: HLA antigen sharing between mother and fetus as a risk factor for eclampsia and pre-eclampsia. *Hum Immunol* 71(3):263–267, 2010.

14. Rugg-Gunn P: Epigenetic features of the mouse trophoblast. *Reprod Biomed Online* 25(1):21–30, 2012.

15. Peixoto AB, Rolo LC, Nardozza LMM, Araujo Júnior E: Epigenetics and pre-eclampsia: Programming of future outcomes. *Methods Mol Biol* 1710:73–83, 2018. doi:10.1007/978-1-4939-7498-6_6.

PART 3

Prediction

7

Prediction of pre-eclampsia

INTRODUCTION

In obstetrics, nothing intrigues one more than the aetiopathology of pre-eclampsia. Despite knowing the deepest and most complicated facets, its exact aetiopathology remains elusive. This gets reflected in the need for its prediction.

CHALLENGES TO TESTS FOR PREDICTION IN PRE-ECLAMPSIA

Many happenings, changes and markers have been identified in the prediction of pre-eclampsia. But which of these are a reflection of the cause or the effect of pre-eclampsia is difficult to identify. The best word that one can use for describing the aetiology and pathology of pre-eclampsia is amorphous. Challenges to prediction methods also come from the inconsistent clinical manifestations of pre-eclampsia besides its amorphous aetiopathology. On one hand, a woman with pre-eclampsia can have a full-blown picture of hypertension, proteinuria and all such. These subjects can have a stillbirth or a growth-retarded foetus. The mother can even have renal failure, vision damage, can throw a fit and can have bleeding diathesis. On the other hand, another woman with pre-eclampsia may just register a rise in blood pressure and sail through the pregnancy without any major complication. This heterogeneity proves a major challenge to the tests of prediction. The clinician wants the tests to predict even the complications of pre-eclampsia. This stretches the tests to a great limit.

One more challenge of this amorphous behaviour of pre-eclampsia is the difference in origin. Pre-eclampsia is at least of two types based on their origin. The pre-eclampsia manifesting at or before 34 weeks has a placental origin, whereas the one manifesting later has a totally different, probably, genetic origin.

NEED FOR MULTIPLE TESTS

In clinical practice, many conditions can be predicted reasonably accurately by a single test. However, pre-eclampsia does not yield to this simplicity. As a result, there is a need for using a combination of tests. Most authorities have used a combination of clinical and biochemical tests. In this list have now been added imaging tests like colour Doppler.

ASSESSING THE QUALITY OF TESTS IN PREDICTION OF PRE-ECLAMPSIA

Prediction of pre-eclampsia has so many tests described in academic literature. This creates the need to judge which tests are reliable. One of the reliable methods for this assessment is scientific review. Another helpful method for judging the efficacy of these tests is computer-based end-user rests. They use binary classifier systems. A receiver operating curve (ROC) is a graphical plot that illustrates the diagnostic ability of a binary classifier system when the discrimination threshold varies as in tests of predicting pre-eclampsia. All these tools are confusing to an average clinician. Even those involved in hard-core research in pre-eclampsia use computer-based tools to use these and to draw valid conclusions. The tests that are going to be included and evaluated in the pages to follow are being so tested with these tools. Valid conclusions are drawn then after to guide the readers.

OVERVIEW OF THE TYPES OF TESTS

Clearly, tests to predict pre-eclampsia can be divided into:

1. Clinical tests,
2. Biochemical tests and
3. Tests based on imaging technology.

A casual look at the list of all tests can show a great disconnect between many of the tests. To illustrate this, what has a Roll-Over Test to do with the assessment of β-hCG? Another example of what has the assessment of soluble Fms-like tyrosine kinase-1 (sFlt-1) to do with colour Doppler of uterine arteries? To a beginner, this may appear like a maze. But, when one delves deep, a profound connection is found between all these tests.

Amongst the clinical tests, there have been many complicated tests proposed. These include the likes of a light-stimulation test. In this, blood pressure changes in the presence of light and darkness is studied. The difference was used to predict pre-eclampsia in a pregnant woman. Thankfully, competent and easier tests have pushed these tests to the throes of research journals.

The biggest group of tests studied are biochemical tests. Some of the biochemical tests are also used in prognostication of the disease. A classic example of this is serum uric acid level estimation. All the chemical substances studied are from diverse families, including hormones, proteins, enzymes, receptors and the like. The list seems to be unending. Estimation of complex biochemical substances never became popular because their efficacy and clinical application remained limited. A classic example of this is the estimation of renin-angiotensin sensitivity test.

Currently, the most popular and apparently, the most efficient amongst all of these are imaging tests. Doppler ultrasound alone or in combination with biochemical markers is currently the most popular test for the prediction of pre-eclampsia.

CLINICAL BEARINGS OF NEGATIVE AND POSITIVE TESTS

There is one important aspect that is quite unique to many of the tests for the prediction of pre-eclampsia. Many of these have excellent negative predictive value. This means that these tests are able to predict that a given pregnant woman has an excellent chance of not developing pre-eclampsia. Most tests in clinical medicine are expected to predict or diagnose a condition positively. However, in pre-eclampsia, even a negative prediction is of great value. It reassures the clinician that the subject will not develop pre-eclampsia.

AN IDEAL TEST

Does idealism exist anywhere? It seems idealism eludes reality. The same holds true for an ideal test to predict pre-eclampsia. For a test to be ideal:

- It should be doable in a clinical setting.
- It should be safe and practical.
- It should not be confined to research and laboratory.
- It should be sensitive and specific.
- Its false-positive rate should be a bare minimum.
- It should be non-invasive.
- It should respect the need and cultural values of the population on which it is performed.

As expected, none of the tests used in predicting pre-eclampsia fit this bill. As a result, it becomes necessary to determine which tests come as close to the ideal as possible.

CLINICAL TESTS

Mid-trimester blood pressure

One of the easiest and probably ancient tests to predict pre-eclampsia is mid-trimester blood pressure. In mid-trimester, in pregnant women without pre-eclampsia, blood pressure tends to fall. Obviously, this fall becomes apparent in women followed serially. This fall can be up to 20 mmHg diastolic. Those pregnant women who did not register a fall have a higher chance of developing pre-eclampsia.

Mean arterial pressure (MAP) was then used because it includes both systolic and diastolic pressure. MAP is calculated as diastolic pressure added to one-third of pulse pressure; 90 was the arbitrary figure considered as a cut-off for the upper limit of permissible pressure. If at mid-trimester on serial estimation, the MAP falls below 90, the pregnant women would not develop pre-eclampsia.

Recently Rocha et al. studied a combination of specified maternal characteristics and MAP in combination to predict pre-eclampsia. They studied this between 11 and 13 weeks. They found a good accuracy in predicting pre-eclampsia.[1]

The roll-over test

The popularity of this test was phenomenal. It is probably the ease with which it can be performed that explains it. Even in busy outdoors and medical college hospital settings in developing countries, it has been performed, studied and extensively documented. It is considered as positive if the subject at mid-trimester is rolled from lateral to supine position, and the blood pressure (diastolic) shows a rise ≥ 20 mmHg. This test has both its good points and not so good points. Interestingly, this test was reported to have great promise about three decades ago. Pregazzi et al. reported a true positive rate of 18.5% and a true negative rate of 88.1%.[2] However, over a period of time, this test fell by the wayside as other studies could not reproduce such impressive results.

Hand-grip test

This is one more clinical test that became popular and has been quite extensively researched and studied. It was also called the "isometric exercise test". It was rated positively when the systolic blood pressure increased by ≥ 15 mmHg during isometric exercise or decreased ≤ 14 mmHg immediately after isometric exercise for a time period of about 30 minutes. This makes it a time-consuming test. More than two decades of study reported high sensitivity (81.8%) and specificity (68.4%) for predicting pregnancy-induced hypertension (PIH) compared to other risk factors.[3] Besides other handicaps, this test like the roll-over test was incompetent for its positive predictive value. This again means that it is good to screen women who will not develop pre-eclampsia, but this is not a good test to predict if women will develop pre-eclampsia. These limitations of the hand-grip test made its use

in clinical practice restricted. As a result, this test is now relegated to the confines of history.

Maternal weight gain in pregnancy

Some old studies showed an association between maternal weight gain in pregnancy and the development of pre-eclampsia. These studies are now archaic and not quoted much.[4] An explanation forwarded for this observation was that early excessive weight gain results in greater maternal fat deposition and inflammation. This, in turn, was postulated to result in hypertension in pregnancy. One relatively recent study has tried to study the association between the development of hypertension in pregnancy and early excessive weight gain. In this study, body mass index (BMI) was also considered along with the weight gain of the subject. It was reported that women whose weight gain exceeded the Institute of Medicine (IOM) guidelines in the first 28 weeks were more likely to develop hypertension in pregnancy even after adjusting for relevant confounders. It was also found that women who were obese had a 2.4-fold increased risk of developing hypertension, even after controlling the confounding variables of weight gain.[5] However, in clinical practice, not much relies upon only weight gain as a sole measure to predict pre-eclampsia.

URINARY TESTS

Microalbuminuria

Amongst tests to predict pre-eclampsia, microalbuminuria became popular in published studies. It occupied a prominent place in literature and journals for some time between the last two decades of the last century and the first few years of this century. Subjects with high levels of microalbuminuria (greater than or equal to 11 mg/mL) were reported to develop pre-eclampsia in up to 83% of cases.[6] Over a period of time, this test was not found to be consistently reliable in predicting pre-eclampsia and therefore, lost popularity. Currently, some sporadic research papers do appear to use this test in combination with other tests for this purpose.[7] Nevertheless, its popularity was highest in the late 1900s.

Besides microalbuminuria, urinary calcium, urinary kallikrein and urinary calcium-to-creatinine ratio have been found to be researched at sometimes or the other to predict pre-eclampsia.

Urinary calcium

Reduced urinary calcium is said to have some association with pre-eclampsia. Besides using it for prediction of pre-eclampsia, hypocalciurea can be used to differentiate between severe pre-eclampsia and chronic hypertension; hypocalciurea is also a marker for disease severity.[8] On the basis of the statistical indices when applied to the results of this test, it has been found that the test is average at best. It had a sensitivity and specificity of 85–90. It has a high negative predictive value. But when the likelihood ratio is applied, urinary hypocalciuric levels (hypocalciurea) remains at best ordinary.[9]

Calcium-to-creatinine ratio

Urinary calcium excretion decreases in pregnancy. There is hypercalciurea in normal pregnancy, which apparently changes in pre-eclampsia. This is the basis of studying urinary calcium-to-creatinine ratio in the prediction of pre-eclampsia. Early studies place 0.066 for calcium-to-creatinine ratio with the use of ROC yielded a sensitivity of 75%, a specificity of 86% and a positive and negative predictive value of 55% and 90%, respectively.[10] Sporadic papers continue to appear in literature thereafter. As late as in 2016, two research papers were cited for this marker in the prediction of pre-eclampsia.[11,12] However, with the onslaught of imaging technology, especially colour Doppler and blood biomarkers, like other urinary tests, calcium-to-creatinine ratio also never became popular in clinical practice.

Kallikrein

Another biochemical marker that has been studied and found some popularity is the excretion of urinary kallikrein. Renal functions have been shown to be significantly affected in pre-eclampsia. This test is believed to reflect the status of renal excretory function. It was with this rationale that urinary kallikrein levels were estimated to predict pre-eclampsia.

In 1996, Miller et al. reported a whopping 83% sensitivity, 91% positivity predictive value and a high likelihood ratio for urinary kallikrein excretion for prediction of pre-eclampsia. In this, they measured urinary kallikrein-to-calcium ratio in a spot urine sample.[13] However, in subsequent studies by others, sensitivity and negative predictive value remained high, but the positive predictive value and specificity were markedly low. Even the likelihood ratio reported in subsequent studies was as low as 3 or even less.[14]

These results, although disproving the hypothesis of renal function compromise as a prerequisite for the onset of clinical pre-eclampsia, also showed an important dissociation. It shows that pre-eclampsia can occur in the absence of compromised renal function. Also, it confirms the thinking that renal involvement is just like any other systemic involvement in pre-eclampsia. It is more an effect of the pathophysiology rather than a part of the aetiopathology of pre-eclampsia.

HAEMATOLOGICAL INDICES

Haematological indices are the most studied and, therefore, constitutes the largest body of prediction tests of PIH in particular. The bunch of these tests and indices includes diverse components. They vary from cellular components of blood like platelets on one end to recent entrants like sFlt-1 on the other end of the spectrum. Many of these are confined to the annals of research journals and laboratory research. Some of these did percolate down to clinical practice.

Cellular components in prediction of pre-eclampsia

LEUCOCYTES

Leucocytes sparingly find a place in some research papers for prediction of pre-eclampsia. A retrospective study of review of records of 33,866 registered births as regards their white blood cell (WBC) count in the first trimester is reported. This study examined if there was a connection between high leucocyte count in the first trimester and development of pre-eclampsia, subsequently. They found an increased risk of preterm delivery but not pre-eclampsia.[15]

PLATELETS AND PLATELET ACTIVATION

Amongst all cellular components, the most conspicuously studied are the platelets. They have been found to have a vital role in sustaining the process of pre-eclampsia in the body of a pregnant woman. Mean platelet volume (MPV) is studied by many research scientists in the prediction of pre-eclampsia. As early as in 1980s platelets have been examined for this purpose. The role of MPV in combination with other markers like uric acid also caught the fascination.[16] It is suggested that MPV progressively increases in women affected by pre-eclampsia as compared with women without pre-eclampsia.[17] These results recurred in some subsequent studies.[18,19] MPV was also tested in sporadic studies in combination with other markers like uric acid, combined Doppler ultrasound, platelet-to-lymphocyte ratio and the like. However, it seems that this marker would never become popular for mass clinical use.

The fundamental reason behind this probing of platelets is the fact that platelet activation plays an important role in the aetiopathology of pre-eclampsia. However, this theoretical basis could never get translated into getting a good and competent platelet-related parameter in the prediction of pre-eclampsia.

URIC ACID

Uric acid estimation in pre-eclampsia is an interesting story. Uric acid was initially thought to have a good role in predicting pre-eclampsia. Uric acid is excreted through kidneys, and so a high level of uric acid meant impaired renal efficiency. This was probably preceding the clinical onset of pre-eclampsia. Delić and Stefanović showed that when parameters such as uric acid (and urea) were included to predict pre-eclampsia based on the multivariate logistic regression model, they could correctly predict it in 79.6% patients.[20] In another complicated statistical analysis, it was found that serum uric acid is a useful test in the management of pre-eclampsia under realistic assumptions.[21] While on uric acid levels, plasma uric acid levels more than 350 μmol/L is thought to be predictive of pre-eclampsia in high-risk subjects.

The popularity of uric acid in pre-eclampsia was not confined to the realms of prediction. It is also a regular entry on the list of "essential" investigations to be carried out in women being managed for pre-eclampsia in many big and small hospitals. It is further amusing that an undergraduate and postgraduate examinee is expected to mention uric acid estimation as an essential investigation when asked to enumerate the list of investigations in a case of pre-eclampsia. All this becomes a little comical. Alterations in uric acid levels are not for diagnosing renal function impairment and the prediction of pre-eclampsia. Uric acid level estimation is more sensitive for the prognosis of pre-eclampsia.

Uric acid is one of the most sensitive reducing systems in the body. Therefore, estimating uric acid is not renal function assessment but more for assessments of oxidative stress that is prevalent. The role of oxidative stress is accepted to be critical in the aetiopathology of obstetric vasculopathies, including pre-eclampsia. Reducing systems like uric acid, therefore, have a significant role to study the process. It is now well-known that reducing systems have a great protective role in the body against oxidative insult. Before oxidative reactive substances react with body tissues and substances, reducing substances react with them and prevent injury.

The policeman-to-riot model to understand the role of uric acid

For better understanding, one can compare the role of uric acid as that of a policeman in preventing riots or trouble in society. During riots, if someone finds that the crew of policemen has remarkably increased over a period of time, it indicates that the situation is grave. It indicates that the riots are not getting under control. So as to combat the rioters, the posse of policemen increases. Thus, more policemen or an increased movement of policemen indicates increased rioting. Applying this to understand the role of uric acid in pre-eclampsia, rising levels of uric acid indicates that "the riot" of oxidative stress has still not been effectively quelled. This means that the process is not coming under effective control. In that case, the prognosis is not good. A rising level of uric acid indicates a poor prognosis. Levels of uric acid expectedly and understandably do not fall until the placenta is out of the body. Until the process and its nidus are not out of the body (foetomaternal interface), the policeman (uric acid) stays put and does not decrease.

In clinical practice, if one finds that the uric acid levels are the same and have not increased remarkably, it means the prognosis is not bad or the situation is not worsening. The maternal reducing systems have been able to effectively stem the disruption. It means that reducing systems production is not increasing anymore. Hence, the estimation of uric acid in a given case of pre-eclampsia should be done for prognostication of the disease and not for diagnosing or screening of the condition.

FIBRONECTIN

Fibronectin is a high-molecular-weight glyco-protein of the extracellular matrix that binds to membrane-spanning receptor proteins called "integrins". Sometimes it serves as a general cell adhesion molecule by anchoring cells to collagen or proteoglycan substrates. Fibronectin is often referred to in the aetiopathology of pre-eclampsia. It became popular in journals for prediction of pre-eclampsia. Besides the prediction of pre-eclampsia, fibronectin has been studied extensively in predicting preterm labour. About two decades ago, some studies appeared that showed that plasma fibronectin levels could represent a specific marker for pre-eclampsia. However, these tests acknowledged that its sensitivity needed to be improved. Its high negative predictive value strongly indicates that the development of pre-eclampsia is less likely in subjects with high levels within the next four weeks after the blood sampling.[22] Aydin et al. showed that elevated maternal plasma fibronectin level above 40 mg/dL is capable of predicting pre-eclampsia with a sensitivity of 73% and a specificity of 92%, suggesting that serial plasma fibronectin measurements before 24 weeks' of gestation may be helpful in the early detection of pre-eclampsia in normotensive gravid women who are destined to become clinically preeclamptic.[23]

It also caught some attention because it was touted to be useful as a single mid-trimester measurement to predict pre-eclampsia in pregnancy. This was, however, summarily disproved. It was found that single mid-trimester assessment of fibronectin levels in maternal plasma was not found to be useful in predicting pre-eclampsia.[24] Series of subsequent studies showed measuring fibronectin to be an unreliable test for predicting pre-eclampsia. Also, a technicality of assessment renders the testing of fibronectin impractical for mass screening. It, therefore, remained confined to journals and reference books on pre-eclampsia

β-hCG

β-hCG has also been used to predict pre-eclampsia. The rationale behind this was that the trophoblastic activity gets reflected in its circulating levels as β-hCG is secreted by the trophoblasts. Levels greater than 2 multiple of median (MOM) at mid-trimester were found to be useful in predicting pre-eclampsia and allied adverse obstetric outcomes.[25] In one of our studies, we found that when low-dose aspirin was given to subjects with raised β-hCG at mid-trimester, adverse obstetric outcomes like miscarriages were reduced and favourable outcomes like full-term deliveries increased.[26]

EPIDEMIOLOGICAL INDICES IN PRE-ECLAMPSIA PREDICTION

Epidemiological indices based on clinical attributes of a pregnant subject are relatively easy to apply. The formal inclusion in a list of recommendations gets labelled as "guidelines". Subsequently, many times algorithms are worked out to guide the clinician on how the clinician has to flow along for diagnosis and management of pre-eclampsia.

One of the most popular and most evaluated guidelines for pre-eclampsia antenatally are the NICE guidelines.[27] These guidelines include the following factors:

1. Hypertensive disorders in previous pregnancy,
2. Chronic kidney disease,
3. Autoimmune disease systemic lupus erythematosus (SLE) or antiphospholipid antibody (APA) syndrome,
4. Type I and II diabetes and
5. Chronic hypertension.

The following were labelled as moderate risk factors:

1. First pregnancy,
2. Age ≥40,
3. Pregnancy interval of more than 10 years,
4. BMI of 35 kg/m^2 at first visit,
5. Family history of pre-eclampsia and
6. Multiple pregnancy.

Nearly all of the high- and moderate-risk factors have been studied individually or in different combinations for prediction of pre-eclampsia. However, they have not proven to be helpful, and so their clinical utility remains limited.

Relatively recently, a model has been suggested that is based on characteristics and medical history for the estimation of patient-specific risk for pre-eclampsia. The authors have suggested that estimation of such a priori risk for pre-eclampsia is an essential first step in the use of Bayes theorem to combine maternal (epidemiological) factors with biomarkers for the continuing development of a more effective method of screening for pre-eclampsia.[28]

Thus, epidemiological indices remain of use in combination with other tests – biochemical or imaging markers in prediction of pre-eclampsia.

COLOUR DOPPLER IN PRE-ECLAMPSIA PREDICTION: THE GAME CHANGER

Ultrasonography is one development in science that changed the face of how obstetrics is practiced. Gone are the days when so much was left to the imagination. X-rays were the only principle imaging modality for medical science until as late as the early 1980s. Students of the subject who have been a witness to the introduction of ultrasonography for widespread use in clinical practice have experienced the joy and ease of diagnosing and managing obstetric situations hitherto left to clinical evaluation and imagination. What began as a non-invasive imaging technique to study the blood supply and its complexities has become a potent weapon for effective prediction, prognostication and decision making in different stages of different obstetric vasculopathies, including pre-eclampsia.

For the prediction of pre-eclampsia, uterine artery colour Doppler is well researched. Uterine arteries can be readily accessed to colour Doppler because it crosses the iliac vessels before entering the uterine musculature and just after giving the cervical (descending) branch. A substantial risk of complications associated with impedance to maternal changes at the level of uterine circulation has been demonstrated.[29,30]

Two forms of changes in the uterine artery are studied: one, changes in Doppler indices pulsatility, resistance and systolic-to-diastolic ratio and second, the diastolic notch in the waveform of the uterine artery for prediction of pre-eclampsia. It was interesting to study the diastolic notch and the behaviour of indices at around 12 weeks and then again at or around mid-trimester. Basically, pulsatility index, resistance index and systolic-to-diastolic ratio help us in identifying the quantum of diastolic flow in the uterine vascular system. This can be better understood if correlated with the pathophysiology occurring at or around this time. The process of the second wave of trophoblastic

invasion is expected to get competently completed at or around mid-trimester. With this moulding, the maternal vascular bed becomes a low-resistance, high-flow pool of blood. It becomes nearly shielded off from the other changes that are taking place in the maternal systems. It also gets shielded off from the pressor substances that may be in circulation in the maternal system at some time or the other. The sum total effect of all these changes is an increase in blood flow to the pregnant uterus. That apart, this increase in blood flow is continuous and guarded by blunting the effects of sympathetic and parasympathetic systems on spiral arterioles.

Review of indices

The commonest indices used in reporting the findings of colour Doppler for the prediction of pre-eclampsia include the resistance index (RI), pulsatility index (PI) and the systolic-to-diastolic ratio (S/D ratio) in the uterine arteries.

In the earlier days of application of colour Doppler in the obstetric world, there was no agreement on the index or a combination of indices to be used for predicting adverse situations of pre-eclampsia. Jacobson et al. used RI for predicting pre-eclampsia. They scanned both uterine arteries at around 20–24 weeks in high-risk subjects for pre-eclampsia. Based on standard deviation, they chose RI of 5.8 as a cut-off. They did not find this index to be reliable enough for predicting pre-eclampsia.[31] Similar results on single measurements of RI at or around mid-trimester were reported by Steel et al.[32] With such dismal results appearing in scientific journals, colour Doppler was nearly given up for predicting pre-eclampsia. However, a later study by Bower et al. revived interest.[33]

More recently, first-trimester uterine artery PI has been shown to be affected by gestational age at screening, maternal weight, racial origin and history of pre-existing diabetes mellitus, and consequently, it should be expressed as MoM after adjustment for these factors. The MoM value of uterine artery PI is significantly increased at 11–13 weeks' gestation in women who subsequently develop pre-eclampsia, and there is a significant negative linear correlation between the PI of the uterine artery with gestational age at delivery.[34] The addition of uterine artery PI to maternal factors improves the detection rates from 36% to 59% and from 33% to 40%, at a false-positive rate of 5%, and from 51% to 75% and from 43% to 55%, at false-positive rate of 10%, for pre-eclampsia requiring delivery before 34 and 37 weeks' gestation, respectively, but not for pre-eclampsia delivering before 42 weeks.[34]

Doppler indices with biomarkers

After this, some biomarkers were used in combination with colour Doppler for the prediction of pre-eclampsia. Florio et al. used alterations in Doppler indices with serum markers like Activin-A and Inhibin-A. They found that the measurement of serum Activin-A and Inhibin-A levels may add significant prognostic information for predicting pre-eclampsia in pregnant women showing specific Doppler alterations late in the second trimester.[35]

Over a period of time, many biomarkers have been used singly or in combination with other markers as well as in combination with uterine artery indices for prediction of pre-eclampsia. The number of markers studied seems to be growing by the day. In a review article published in 2015, a total of six biomarker algorithms, for the prediction of pre-eclampsia were studied. Several algorithms were based on placental biomarkers such as pregnancy-associated plasma protein A (PAPP-A), placental growth factor (PlGF) and s-FLT-1. The algorithms containing these biomarkers showed a high prediction rate for early onset PE, ranging from 44% to 92% at 5% false-positive rate. New biomarkers suggest an alternative model based on free foetal haemoglobin (HbF) and the heme scavenger alpha-1-microglobulin (A1M) with a prediction rate of 69% at an false-positive rate of 5%. They found that this model performs well even without uterine artery Doppler PI.[36]

The current guideline from NICE is used extensively and popularly for the prediction of pre-eclampsia. It recommends that, at the booking visit, women identified with one major risk factor or more than one moderate risk factor for pre-eclampsia should be advised to take low-dose aspirin daily from 12 weeks until delivery. However, the performance of this method of screening is poor and identifies only about 35% of pre-eclampsia.[37] Currently, the National Health Service (NHS) group in England is working on a protocol for the prospective validation study, which they call as "Screening Programme for Pre-Eclampsia" (SPREE). While announcing this study, this group states that the best performance for early prediction of pre-eclampsia can be achieved by using a novel method based on Bayes' theorem that combines maternal characteristics and medical history together with measurements of MAP, uterine artery pulsatility index (UtA-PI), serum PlGF and PAPP-A at 11–13 weeks' gestation. Eligible pregnant women attending their routine scan at 11–13 weeks' gestation are invited to participate in this study. This forms the "combined test", which could be simplified to the "mini combined test" when only maternal factors, MAP and PAPP-A are taken into consideration. Maternal characteristics and history and measurements of MAP, UtA-PI, serum PAPP-A and PlGF are recorded according to standardised protocols. The patient-specific risk for pre-eclampsia will be calculated and data on pregnancy outcomes collected. They begin their study with the hypothesis that the first-trimester mini combined test and combined test, for pre-eclampsia screening, using the method based on Bayes' theorem, are likely to be superior to the current method recommended by NICE that is based on maternal demographics and history alone. Enrolment for the study commenced in April 2016.[37] This study will in most likelihood confirm the efficacy of a combination of maternal characteristics and history, clinical measurements of MAP and biomarkers in the prediction of pre-eclampsia.

The diastolic notch

As a part of a routine second trimester obstetric scan, a good imaging spectrum always includes a mention of the presence or otherwise of diastolic notch in the uterine artery.

What is diastolic notch?

At 12–14 weeks of duration of normal pregnancy, the uterine artery consistently shows the presence of a diastolic notch as shown in Figure 7.1. This is the small dip found just before the diastolic wave begins as mentioned. The presence of diastolic notch suggests that the second wave of trophoblastic invasion is still not complete. It suggests that the process may be ongoing but is still

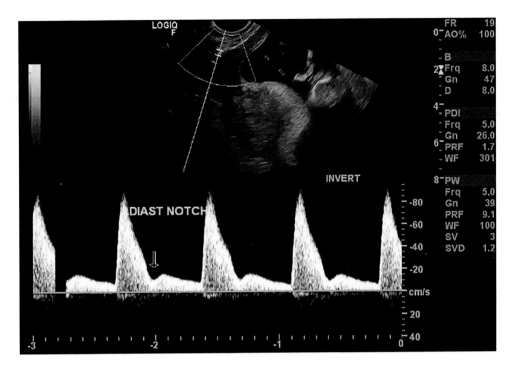

Figure 7.1 Diastolic notch.

not over. The presence of diastolic notch in these subjects at 12–14 weeks may not have much significance except indicating that the process is ongoing. The disappearance of the diastolic notch seems to be a reliable predictor of obstetric vasculopathy. This occurs at around mid-trimester or then after any time.

Chan et al. showed that the combination of a diastolic notch and an abnormal RI in both uterine arteries at 20 weeks' gestation is the most accurate indicator in predicting severe pregnancy complications. These subjects are almost eight times more likely to develop clinically significant hypertension, delivery prior to 34 weeks, have a perinatal demise or have an infant with a birth weight <1,500 g.[38]

Over a period of time, the absence of diastolic notch as shown in Figure 7.2 or its disappearance seems to be a popular predictor of obstetric vasculopathies especially of pre-eclampsia and IUGR. Besides reviving interest in colour Doppler in the prediction of pre-eclampsia, Bower et al. used the disappearance of the diastolic notch to predict pre-eclampsia.[33] They found a higher sensitivity and positive predictive value in the disappearance of the diastolic notch for predicting pre-eclampsia.

Additionally, this study used a two-stage test. They studied the subjects first at 18–22 weeks of pregnancy, and then they studied them again at 24 weeks and found the disappearance of the diastolic notch to be a good predictor of pre-eclampsia. This has been conclusively proven in other subsequent studies.[39,40]

Practical problem with using colour Doppler and biomarker in combination

Most of the studies in the prediction of pre-eclampsia have proven beyond a doubt that a combination of tests is always better job. As a result, studies emerging from countries like the United States and the United Kingdom (UK) use a combination of imaging and biomarker tests for this purpose. This is reproduced throughout the world, including countries like India. However, none of these tests pay heed to an important practical problem – who will pay for these tests? In the UK, for example, from where a big body of these studies has been published, it is usually the NHS that pays for the tests. They are a part of universal screening for chromosomal anomalies like Trisomy-21 of all pregnant mothers. In India, on the

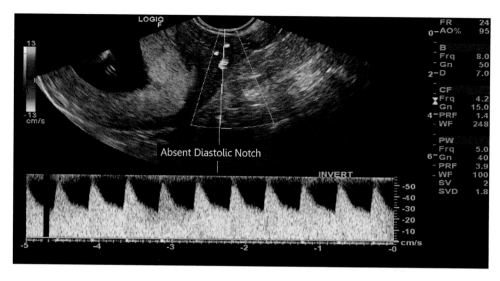

Figure 7.2 Absent diastolic notch.

other hand, the situation is completely different. Here the tests have to be paid for by the pregnant woman from her personal resources. As a part of the normal practice, in India, all pregnant women who get a reasonably good quality of antenatal care, are subjected to 11–13 weeks ultrasound scan. It is at this scan that the colour Doppler of the uterine artery is also done. In subjects who are older than 35 years of age, have a high-risk factor in their history, or in soft-markers are then after subjected to a biomarker test like PAPP-A and others. The number of women who are thus subjected to a double set of screening tests is low. Insisting on the use of biomarkers for pre-eclampsia screening in this type of practice increases the financial burden for the family. Therefore, there is a need to examine the possibility of eliminating one of the sets of these tests, either sonography or biomarkers.

This has been found to be possible by using two markers on a ultrasound scan at 11–13 weeks of pregnancy. Our group has been involved in exploring this possibility. We first examined the efficacy of PI > 1.7 alone in the prediction of pre-eclampsia: 489 pregnant women with singleton pregnancies were prospectively studied. It was found that PI > 1.7 alone was quite efficient in predicting pre-eclampsia. Its χ^2 value was 0.004, which was significant at $P < 0.05$. It had good sensitivity and specificity with a 95% confidence interval (CI). It had a positive predictive value of 10.53% and a negative predictive value of 80.17%. We combined PI with another ultrasound marker – notch depth index.

Notch Depth Index

A quantitative index – the notch depth index (NDI) – has been developed and evaluated for its association with the risk of obstetric vasculopathies like pre-eclampsia and a SGA infant. It is calculated as the depth of the diastolic notch divided by the maximal diastolic velocity as shown in Figure 7.3.

Ohkuchi et al. evaluated the association of the NDI with the risk of pre-eclampsia and a SGA infant and to compare its clinical usefulness with that of the uterine artery RI and the peak S/D ratio. They studied in 288 consecutive healthy pregnant subjects at 20.2 ± 2.0 (range 16.0–23.9) weeks of gestation and found that the NDI value in the second trimester is associated with the later onset of pre-eclampsia and is clinically more useful in predicting pre-eclampsia than the two conventional indices.[41]

We used this NDI in combination with PI > 1.7 and evaluated the efficacy of this combination in the prediction of pre-eclampsia. In all, 228 pregnant women had such a combination of PI > 1.7 and NDI > 0.5. It was found that their chance of developing pre-eclampsia was highly significant with a χ^2 value of 22.8233 ($P < 0.05$). The sensitivity and specificity of this combination were within 95% CI.[42]

Without the need for a biomarker, only from the scan from the first trimester it was possible to use two sets of parameters and get satisfactory and valid results for prediction of pre-eclampsia.

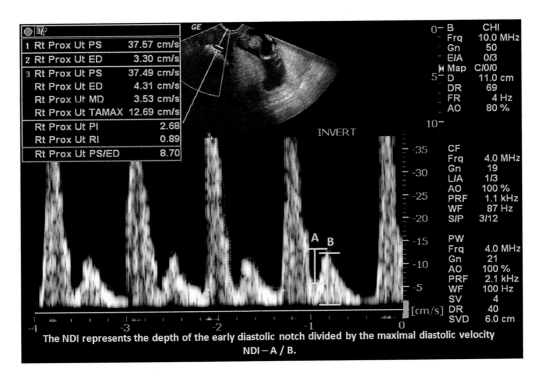

The NDI represents the depth of the early diastolic notch divided by the maximal diastolic velocity
NDI – A / B.

Figure 7.3 Notch depth index (NDI).

This eliminated the need for using biomarkers in the prediction of pre-eclampsia without compromising on the quality of results. Uterine artery colour Doppler can be made to work still harder in pre-eclampsia prediction.

Doppler indices for the discontinuation of preventive measures

While these attempts are ongoing, PI alone was studied for its efficacy in predicting pre-eclampsia. PI > 1.7 has been consistently reported to be indicative of high risk for the development of pre-eclampsia. On the other hand, PI < 1 as an isolated marker was found to be effective in predicting low-risk subjects for pre-eclampsia. It was found that those subjects with a PI < 1 in the second trimester have significantly fewer chances of developing pre-eclampsia. Many times in clinical practice, aspirin is started on the basis of history. In such subjects, PI < 1 could help in stopping preventive measures.[43] To reinforce this parameter, we also studied a combination of PI < 1.0 and absent diastolic notch in the first trimester. There were 110 such subjects in

our study with PI < 1.0 and absent diastolic notch in the first trimester. They were found to be at low risk for developing pre-eclampsia. The P value for this test was 0.002 which was highly significant. With a good sensitivity and specificity at 95% CI, this test had a false-positive rate of less than 5%.[43]

If on the basis of colour Doppler, women who had a risk of developing pre-eclampsia show on a subsequent scan that the risk is now low, obstetricians can discontinue preventive measures like aspirin or aspirin and heparin combination. For this, uterine artery colour Doppler requires to be repeated again in the second trimester (about 20 weeks) at the time of targeted scan for congenital anomalies. If that subject who showed a presence of uterine artery in the first trimester shows its persistence of diastolic notch in the second trimester, her chances of developing pre-eclampsia are still high. The preventive measures should not be discontinued. We prospectively studied 451 women, and in 57 of these, the diastolic notch persisted in the second trimester. Highly significant subjects developed pre-eclampsia with P < 0.01. This finding had a high specificity of 84.77%, a negative predictive value of 90.03% and a high accuracy (Unpublished data).

Identifying low-risk subjects in the first trimester

Usually, uterine artery scans in the first trimester are used for identifying women at high risk for pre-eclampsia. Stretching the use of colour Doppler still further, we found that not only is this technology efficient in predicting women at high risk for developing pre-eclampsia, it can also identify those at low risk. For this, we used two parameters: PI < 1.0 and absent diastolic notch in uterine artery scans in the first trimester. As such, we prospectively followed 510 subjects that met the criteria and found that they had a significant low risk of developing pre-eclampsia. The difference was statistically highly significant with a low P value (unpublished data). Thus, over a period of time, uterine artery colour Doppler has become the most reliable and versatile technology in the prediction of pre-eclampsia.

THE FUTURE: NANOPARTICLES INCLUDING EXOSOMES

One of the most promising area for the future in identifying the aetiology and subsequently in prediction of pre-eclampsia is the area of placenta-derived extracellular vesicles in general and exosomes in particular. These nanoparticles, and probably infra-nanoparticles, in circulation are being studied closely these days for their role in various conditions from malignancy to obstetric conditions like pre-eclampsia and gestational diabetes mellitus. With such a wide-ranging field of focus, the picture is likely to be confusing. The term "extracellular vesicle" is nonspecific, and it includes all membrane-bound vesicles from nanometre to micrometre diameters and of different origins. Currently, there is a lack of standardised nomenclature of these particles. This also contributes to the prevailing confusing picture. So as to confidently attribute some particular function to these tiny vesicles, lots of specificity in their characterisation will be required.

There are some areas on which there is an agreement. First, exosomes are a subtype of extracellular vesicles with a particle size (40–120 nm) and density (1.13–1.19 g/mL^{-1}). Exosomes have an interesting cargo that they carry. They are specifically packaged with signalling molecules (including protein, messenger RNA, microRNA and noncoding RNA). They are released from the cells by the process of exocytosis into various biofluid compartments. They are taken into the target cells by the process of endocytosis. Exosomes can regulate the activity of its target cells. For understanding their role in pre-eclampsia and their role in activities like angiogenesis, cellular proliferation and apoptosis are of interest.

Basically exosomes are signalling particles, which establish a communication line between maternal and foetal cells. Current techniques are able to identify the exosomes of placental origin at 6 weeks. However, with the establishment of enough evidence for the physiology of foetomaternal crosstalk within days of fertilisation and implantation, it will be possible to establish their presence even before 6 weeks of pregnancy.

Oxygen or lack of it (anaerobic environment) is essential for initial successful implantation and good quality and successful foetomaternal crosstalk. The entire activity of uterine glands, uterine milk and some obstetric complications have their basis early in the days of pregnancy. It has been found that oxygen is critical for the release of exosomes. Both these events are occurring early in pregnancy and are likely to be interrelated. Glucose is one more molecule that has been identified to be critical in the release of exosomes. With science currently examining the role of exosomes in pre-eclampsia, it is safe to assume that the roots of this condition in particular and other obstetric vasculopathies in general are laid early in pregnancy. Immune tolerance is a function of exosomes. At the heart of obstetric vasculopathies lies the disturbance in immune tolerance. The role of exosomes in the aetiology of these conditions is therefore important. The functions of placental exosomes in pregnancy are still to be uncovered completely.

It seems the extracellular microvesicles – exosomes – are released by the syncitiotrophoblasts. They establish the communication line between the mother and the foetus. Successful and robust foetomaternal communication ensures healthy placentation. A healthy placentation subsequently leads to a healthy pregnancy outcome preventing placenta-based disorders – the obstetric vasculopathies. Here begins the complexity.

Syncitiotrophoblasts have been identified specifically in many different states that cause oxidative stress at the foetomaternal interface as well as the entire maternal endothelial bed. This oxidative stress causes pre-eclampsia as has been elaborated elsewhere in this book. These extracellular vesicles, termed "syncytiotrophoblast microvesicles", may bind to monocytes and stimulate the production of proinflammatory cytokines. This in turn results in altered maternal systemic inflammatory response in normal and pre-eclamptic pregnancies.[44–47] Some interesting studies from the UK have shown that exosomes may be a key constituent of syncytiotrophoblast microvesicles involved in the pathogenesis of the disorder.[45,47–51]

The proposed mechanism behind the role played by exosomes in the causation of pre-eclampsia is interesting. Understanding this mechanism helps further in using the exosomes in predicting pre-eclampsia. Subsequently, this may also hold the promise of devising the treatment of pre-eclampsia. Exosomes are the key constituents of exocellular vesicles released by syncitiotrophoblasts. This is because of their ability to reprogram cells and subsequently alter the normal physiology and activities of the cells. This in turn contributes to many pathological conditions. Basically, exosomes are the communication medium through which foetoplacental crosstalk takes place. The syncitiotrophoblasts package the exosomes with genetic and proteomic information. This is carried by the exosomes to the target cells where the decoding takes place. This results in a series of changes that can cause different obstetric vasculopathies, including pre-eclampsia. If a system gets developed wherein the exosomes carrying this disease-creating information is decoded well before their clinical manifestations, the exosomes can help in prediction of these conditions. In that case, it is likely that exosomes would be the most specific marker of pre-eclampsia and other obstetric vasculopathies like IUGR. Also, manipulating these genetic signals through stem cells or by any other method holds promise to the treatment of pre-eclampsia.

Currently, it is wisely asked if exosomes can be objectively isolated, detected and quantified from biological fluids. Have they been shown to increase with an increase in gestational age in normal pregnancy? Have they been shown to be significantly altered in pre-eclampsia? Do they contain key molecular markers that can improve biomarker sensitivity and specificity? Can they be used as a biotherapeutic agent to reprogram the dysfunctional placenta?[52] Though this is futuristic, herein probably lies the key.

REFERENCES

1. Rocha RS, Alves JAG, Maia E Holanda Moura SB, Araujo Júnior E, Peixoto AB, Santana EFM, Martins WP et al.: Simple approach based on maternal characteristics and mean arterial pressure for the prediction of preeclampsia in the first trimester of pregnancy. *J Perinat Med* 45(7):843–849, 2017. doi:10.1515/jpm-2016-0418.
2. Pregazzi R, Levi D'Ancona R, Venuleo V, Scrimin F, Ricci G, Toffoletti FG, Barciulli F: Prediction of EPH gestosis by means of the roll-over test, clinical contribution. *Minerva Ginecol* 43(12):545–548, 1991.
3. Tomoda S, Kitanaka T, Ogita S, Hidaka A: Prediction of pregnancy-induced hypertension by isometric exercise. *Asia Oceania J Obstet Gynaecol* 20(3):249–255, 1994.
4. Gardiner J, Herdan G: A statistical evaluation of the nitroglycerine flicker-fusion threshold test and the weight-gain sign in the prediction of the clinical syndrome of pre-eclampsia. *J Obstet Gynaecol Br Emp* 64(5):691–699, 1957.
5. Ruhstaller KE, Bastek JA, Thomas A, Mcelrath TF, Parry SI, Durnwald CP: The effect of early excessive weight gain on the development of hypertension in pregnancy. *Am J Perinatol* 33(12):1205–1210, 2016. doi:10.1055/s-0036-1585581.
6. Rodriguez MH, Masaki DI, Mestman J, Kumar D, Rude R: Calcium/creatinine ratio and microalbuminuria in the prediction of preeclampsia. *Am J Obstet Gynecol* 159(6):1452–1455, 1988.
7. Chen H, Zhang J, Qin F, Chen X, Jiang X: Evaluation of the predictive value of high sensitivity C-reactive protein in pregnancy-induced hypertension syndrome. *Exp Ther Med* 16(2):619–622, 2018. doi:10.3892/etm.2018.6246.
8. Friedman S, Lindheimer S: Prediction and differential diagnosis. In Lindheimer M, Roberts J, Cunningham F, editors: *Chesley, Hypertensive Disorders of Pregnancy*, 2nd ed., pp. 201–228, 1998, Stamford, CT, Appleton & Lange.
9. Henderson JT, Thompson JH, Burda BU, Cantor A, Beil T, Whitlock EP: Screening for preeclampsia: A systematic evidence

review for the U.S. preventive services task Force [Internet]. U.S. Preventive Services Task Force Evidence Syntheses, formerly systematic evidence reviews. Rockville, MD: Agency for Healthcare Research and Quality (US); April 2017. Report No.: 14-05211-EF-1.

10. Ozcan T, Kaleli B, Ozeren M, Turan C, Zorlu G: Urinary calcium to creatinine ratio for predicting preeclampsia. *Am J Perinatol* 12(5):349–351, 1995.

11. David A, Padmaja P: Calcium-to-creatinine ratio in a spot sample of urine, for early prediction of hypertensive disorders of pregnancy: A prospective study. *J Obstet Gynaecol India* 66(Suppl 1):94–97, 2016. doi: 10.1007/s13224-015-0797-3.

12. Munge A, Satia M: Urinary calcium to creatinine ratio to predict preeclampsia and use of calcium supplementation to prevent preeclampsia. *Int Jr Reprod Contraception Obstet Gynecol* 5(5):1380–1385, 2017.

13. Millar J, Campbell S, Albano J, Higgins B, Clark A: Early prediction of preeclampsia by measurement of kallikrein and creatinine on a random urine sample. *Br J Obstet Gynecol* 103(5):421–426, 1996.

14. Kyle P, Campbell S, Buckley D, Kissane J, de Swiet M, Albano J, Millar J, Redman C: A comparison of the inactive urinary kallikrein: Creatinine ratio and the angiotensin sensitivity test for the prediction of preeclampsia. *Br J Obstet Gynecol* 103(10):981–987, 1996.

15. Tzur T, Weintraub AY, Sergienko R, Sheiner E: Can leukocyte count during the first trimester of pregnancy predict later gestational complications? *Arch Gynecol Obstet* 287(3):421–427, 2013. doi:10.1007/s00404-012-2603-0.

16. Fay RA, Bromham DR, Brooks JA, Gebski VJ: Platelets and uric acid in the prediction of preeclampsia. *Am J Obstet Gynecol* 152(8):1038–1039, 1985.

17. Dundar O, Yoruk P, Tutuncu L, Erikci AA, Muhcu M, Ergur AR, Atay V, Mungen E: Longitudinal study of platelet size changes in gestation and predictive power of elevated MPV in development of preeclampsia. *Prenat Diagn* 28(11):1052–1056, 2008. doi:10.1002/pd.2126.

18. Kashanian M, Hajjaran M, Khatami E, Sheikhansari N: Evaluation of the value of the first and third trimester maternal mean platelet volume (MPV) for prediction of pre-eclampsia. *Pregnancy Hypertens* 3(4):222–226, 2013. doi:10.1016/j.preghy.2013.06.001.

19. Kanat-Pektas M, Yesildager U, Tuncer N, Arioz DT, Nadirgil-Koken G, Yilmazer M: Could mean platelet volume in late first trimester of pregnancy predict intrauterine growth restriction and pre-eclampsia? *J Obstet Gynaecol Res* 40(7):1840–1845, 2014. doi:10.1111/jog.12433.

20. Delić R, Stefanović M: Optimal laboratory panel for predicting preeclampsia. *J Matern Fetal Neonatal Med* 23(1):96–102, 2010.

21. Koopmans C, van Pampus M, Groen H, Aarnoudse J, van den Berg P, Mol BW: Accuracy of serum uric acid as a predictive test for maternal complications in preeclampsia: Bivariate meta-analysis and decision analysis. *Eur J Obstet Gynecol Reprod Biol* 146(1):8–14, 2009.

22. Dreyfus M, Baldauf JJ, Ritter J, Van Cauwenberg JR, Hardy A, Foidart JM: The prediction of preeclampsia: Reassessment of clinical value of increased plasma levels of fibronectin. *Eur J Obstet Gynecol Reprod Biol* 78(1):25–28, 1998.

23. Aydin T, Varol F, Sayin N: Third trimester maternal plasma total fibronectin levels in pregnancy-induced hypertension: Results of a tertiary center. *Clin Appl Thromb Hemost* 12(1):33–39, 2006.

24. Ajibola SO, Adeyemo TA, Afolabi BB, Akanmu AS: Utility of a single mid-trimester measurement of plasminogen activator Type 1 and fibronectin to predict preeclampsia in pregnancy. *Niger Med J* 57(4):213–216, 2016. doi:10.4103/0300-1652.188337.

25. Desai P, Rao S: Predictive value of raised midtrimester HCG in P.I.H. *J Obstet Gynaecol India* 52(1):68–70, 2002.

26. Desai P, Rao S: Role of low dose aspirin in mothers registering high serum HCG levels at mid trimester. *J Obstet Gynaecol India* 52(5):30–32, 2002.

27. National Collaborating Centre for Women's and Children's Health. Hypertension in pregnancy.

The management of hypertensive disorders during pregnancy. Clinical guideline no. 107. London, National Institute for Health and Clinical Excellence, 2010.

28. Wright D, Syngelaki A, Akolekar R, Poon LC, Nicolaides KH: Competing risks model in screening for preeclampsia by maternal characteristics and medical history. *Am J Obstet Gynecol* 213(1):62.e1–62.e10, 2015. doi:10.1016/j.ajog.2015.02.018.

29. Hernandez-Andrade E, Brodzki J, Lingman G: Uterine artery score and perinatal outcome. *Ultrasound Obstet Gynecol* 19:438, 2002.

30. Lees C, Para M, Missfelder Lobos H: Individualized risk assessment for adverse pregnancy outcome by uterine artery Doppler at 23 weeks. *Obstet Gynecol* 98: 369, 2001.

31. Jacobson S, Inhofe R, Manning N: The value of Doppler assessment at the uteroplacental circulation in predicting preeclampsia and IUGR. *Am J Obstet Gynecol* 162: 110–114, 1990.

32. Steel S, Pearce J, Mc Parland P, Chamberlain G: Early Doppler ultrasound screening in prediction of hypertensive disorders of pregnancy. *Lancet* 335: 1548–1551, 1990.

33. Bower S, Bewley S, Campbell S: Improved prediction of preeclampsia by two-stage screening of uterine arteries using the early diastolic notch and colour Doppler imaging. *Obstet Gynecol* 82:78–83, 1994.

34. Wright D, Akolekar R, Syngelaki A, Poon LC, Nicolaides KH: A competing risks model in early screening for preeclampsia. *Fetal Diagn Ther* 32:171–178, 2012.

35. Florio P, Reis F, Pezzani I, Luisi S, Severi F, Petraglia F: The addition of Activin A and inhibin A measurement to uterine artery Doppler velocimetry to improve the early prediction of preeclampsia. *Ultrasound Obstet Gynecol* 21(2):165–169, 2003.

36. Anderson UD, Gram M, Åkerström B, Hansson SR: First trimester prediction of preeclampsia. *Curr Hypertens Rep* 17(9):584, 2015. doi:10.1007/s11906-015-0584-7.

37. Tan MY, Koutoulas L, Wright D, Nicolaides KH, Poon LCY: Protocol for the prospective validation study: "Screening programme for pre-eclampsia" (SPREE). *Ultrasound Obstet Gynecol* 50(2):175–179, 2017. doi:10.1002/uog.17467.

38. Chan FY, Pun TC, Lam C et al.: Pregnancy screening by uterine artery Doppler velocimetry – Which criterion performs the best. *Obstet Gynecol* 85:696–602, 1995.

39. Phupong V, Dejthevaporn T: Predicting risks of preeclampsia and small for gestational age infant by uterine artery Doppler. *Hypertens Pregnancy* 27(4):387–395, 2008.

40. Hafner E, Metzenbauer M, Höfinger D, Stonek F, Schuchter K, Waldhör T, Philipp K: Comparison between three-dimensional placental volume at 12 weeks and uterine artery impedance/notching at 22 weeks in screening for pregnancy-induced hypertension, preeclampsia and fetal growth restriction in a low-risk population. *Ultrasound Obstet Gynecol* 27(6):652–657, 2006.

41. Ohkuchi A, Minakami H, Sato I, Mori H, Nakano T, Tateno M: Predicting the risk of preeclampsia and a small-for-gestational-age infant by quantitative assessment of the diastolic notch in uterine artery flow velocity waveforms in unselected women. *Ultrasound Obstet Gynecol* 16(2):171–178, 2000.

42. Desai P: Notch depth index alone and in combination with PI in prediction of preeclampsia at or before 32 weeks of pregnancy. *Pregnancy Hypertens* 16:11–15, 2019.

43. Desai P, Desai M: Uterine artery pulsatility index less than 1.0 as an isolated marker in predicting low-risk subjects for preeclampsia. *Int J Reprod Contraception Obstet Gynecol* 5(5):1300–1303, 2016.

44. Redman CW, Sargent IL: Microparticles and immunomodulation in pregnancy and pre-eclampsia. *J Reprod Immunol* 76:61–67, 2007.

45. Redman CW, Sargent IL: Pre-eclampsia, the placenta and the maternal systemic inflammatory response: A review. *Placenta* 24:S21–S27, 2003.

46. Sargent IL, Germain SL, Sacks GP, Kumar S, Redman CW: Trophoblast deportation and the maternal inflammatory response in pre-eclampsia. *J Reprod Immunol* 59:153–160, 2003.

47. Germain SJ, Sacks GP, Sooranna SR, Sargent IL, Redman CW: Systemic inflammatory priming in normal pregnancy and preeclampsia: The role of circulating syncytiotrophoblast microparticles. *J Immunol* 178:5949–5956, 2007.

48. Redman CW, Sargent IL: Placental debris, oxidative stress and pre-eclampsia. *Placenta* 21:597–602, 2000.

49. Southcombe J, Tannetta D, Redman C, Sargent I: The immunomodulatory role of syncytiotrophoblast microvesicles. *PLoS One* 6:e20245, 2011.

50. Tannetta D, Masliukaite I, Vatish M, Redman C, Sargent I: Update of syncytiotrophoblast derived extracellular vesicles in normal pregnancy and preeclampsia. *J Reprod Immunol* 119:98–106, 2017.

51. Tannetta D, Collett G, Vatish M, Redman C, Sargent I: Syncytiotrophoblast extracellular vesicles: Circulating biopsies reflecting placental health. *Placenta* 52:134–138, 2017.

52. Pillay P, Moodley K, Moodley J, Mackraj I: Placenta-derived exosomes: Potential biomarkers of preeclampsia. *Int J Nanomedicine* 12:8009–8023, 2017. doi:10.2147/IJN.S142732.

PART **4**

Prevention

8

Prevention of pre-eclampsia

INTRODUCTION

Dying, they say, will be optional when the aging process is reversible, according to genetic engineers. Corden'o and Wood published *The Death of Death* and have postulated that by 2045 CE, death will be optional. Until that time that this situation becomes a possibility on a mass scale, clinicians and research scientists have to combat disease conditions whose causes are still illusory.

In obstetrics, the main condition that alludes an accurate explanation for its cause is pre-eclampsia. For us, therefore, the prevention of pre-eclampsia is a big focus area. If one cannot treat the cause, then treat its effects – that is a common and wide practice in modern medical science. This applies to pre-eclampsia as well. Preventive measures, therefore, rely more on prevention of manifestations.

WHAT IS THE DIFFERENCE BETWEEN DISEASE AND DERANGEMENT?

The basic difference between disease and derangment is in the body response. The body response to a disease state is usually decisive and tends to stem the disease process. In derangements, the body response is relatively subdued and becomes energetic only when the condition heavily worsens. As a result, treatment measures can provide inconsistent responses in derangements. On the other hand, the body responds to diseases inconsistently. This seems to result from the perception of derangement by the body as its innate process and the disease as an attack on itself. The difference between disease and derangement has been extensively discussed the first time in 2013.[1]

It would be easier to understand this through examples. Malignancies are considered derangements and malaria, a disease. Malignancies anywhere in the body do not incite an immediate response on occurrence. They tend to run an insidious course with the body's protective mechanisms trying to handle and suppress the conditions. They, therefore, grow gradually and hardly produce any clinical features. It is, therefore, said in euphemism that malignancies usually do not cause pain and a painful mass is usually not malignant. On the other hand, the body responds torridly to malaria. Fever with rigor, headache, generalised body ache and a similar series of clinical features develop. It is produced by an exogenous element – the malarial parasite and, therefore, is perceived as foreign by the human body. Malignancies, atherosclerosis and, along similar lines, obstetric vasculopathies are not perceived as foreign by the human body. They are a part of its own for the body. Therefore, the response of the body to these is muted and insidious. The features that occur are only of the complications and systemic effects of these derangements.

There is still more to this. By understanding the difference between derangement and disease, one can predict if these conditions will be cured or will be controlled. Diseases get cured, and derangements get controlled. Nutritional anaemia in pregnancy is a disease. It can be cured by administering the nutritional hemopoietic substance. On the other hand, non-nutritional anaemia resulting from sickle cell disease or thalassemia is a derangement. Therefore, these conditions cannot be cured. They can either be controlled or if the entire marrow is replaced can be changed, but they cannot be cured. Diabetes too is a derangement. It is a derangement of insulin production, activity and metabolism. The basic cause is insulin deficiency which may be genetic or age acquired. Therefore, diabetes can be controlled, but it cannot be cured. Diabetes is, therefore, not a disease it is a derangement.

On the other hand, viral hepatitis seemingly has no cure. But from medical science, it is a known viral disease. Once the viral load is overwhelmed by the body's resistance mechanisms, the disease gets cured. Like anaemia, jaundice can also be a derangement. Types of liver derangements, which result from factors that produce a permanent dysfunction of liver function as in hepatitis C are derangements. They elude a cure. A liver transplant replaces the dead liver tissue by a healthy and functioning new hepatic tissue. But that is not a cure for the original disease. It is just a circumvention of the diseased system.

Why is this differentiation so important? Scientists in search of immortality continue to find cures for derangements. Cures that never existed can never be created. Derangements are incurable. They can be controlled, their complications prevented and their progress thwarted but they cannot be cured. If diseases can be cured, then derangements can be controlled. Atherosclerosis causing a disease like myocardial infarction may be preventable, but the derangement of atherosclerosis cannot be cured.

This does not mean that the difference between a disease and a derangement is always watertight. It can also get blurred. In the initial stages, derangements can be transiently reversed or their progress slowed and worsening postponed. But the process continues to lurk at the cellular level. It can strike again because there is no cure. A regular follow-up and surveillance is needed for early diagnosis of a deterioration. One interesting point comes up here regarding the progress of cervical intraepithelial neoplasia (CIN). The CIN-1 can progress to CIN-II and get reversed. But once CIN-III occurs, it becomes irreversible. Gynaecologists may then use fanciful names of removing the lesion by cone biopsy or loop excision or even hysterectomy. But they cannot cure or reverse it. In early stages, therefore, the condition gets cured. As soon as the cervical junction gets deranged permanently, it starts producing cells that are malignant or potentially malignant. Now at this stage, this condition cannot be cured.

Can stem cells cure a derangement? The answer technically is no. Stem cells act by marrow replacement in leukaemia or thalassemia. It replaces the deranged manufacturing line. It generates a different and new line that is healthy and competent. Clinically, patients will be free of the condition but technically they were not "cured". The dysfunctional system was not restored to regain its function. Therefore, even stem cells will not be able to "treat" a derangement; they will only replace the derangement by healthy systems.

Having had known and understood this difference well, it can now be understood why the treatment of pre-eclampsia, in particular, is not found. Obstetric vasculopathies like pre-eclampsia are derangements. They cannot be cured. They can be controlled. They can be prevented from worsening. Their complications can be prevented. But the parent condition cannot be cured.

In a greatly dramatized mention, Lindheimer et al. photographed and inserted it in their book *Chesley's Hypertensive Disorders of Pregnancy* a picture of placards honouring famous physicians who have made major contributions to the field of obstetrics. This placard holder stands at Chicago Lying-In Hospital. They point at an empty plaque, which they say is reserved for a person who discovers the cause and cure for pre-eclampsia. This plaque is reportedly still empty.[2] If the custodians of this plaque holder are and shall remain honest to the causes and purpose of erecting it, the plaque for the person finding the cause and cure of pre-eclampsia will remain vacant for all eternity. This is because there is no cure for pre-eclampsia. Pre-eclampsia is not a disease. Pre-eclampsia is a derangement. It will never reveal its cause. It will never get cured. It can be controlled. It can be prevented from worsening and its complications can be prevented or kept to a bare minimum. But a cure does not exist. Derangements do not get cured. Once humanity accepts this limitation of its existence, the struggle and needless useless attempts shall become relegated to history. It is possible that staring at this empty plaque for decades, its custodians may finally compromise and insert the name of the person who described its aetiopathology. But if they want the name of the person who cures it or tells us what causes it, the plaque is destined to remain empty.

WHICH SUBJECTS MAY BENEFIT?

Those women who are at a high risk of developing pre-eclampsia are the ones that should benefit from preventive measures. But the bigger question is that which pregnant women are at a high risk? A history of an adverse outcome can provide vital clues of a woman at risk of obstetric vasculopathies including pre-eclampsia. Anyone or more than one manifestation of obstetric vasculopathies like pre-eclampsia remote from term or recurrent missed abortion late in the first trimester or early second trimester, intrauterine growth restriction (IUGR), accidental haemorrhage and the like are some of the conditions, which can make a subject vulnerable to a recurrence of obstetric vasculopathies. The same obstetric vasculopathy does not need to recur. It may be pre-eclampsia remote from term in one pregnancy and the other time she can have an IUGR. Nevertheless, women with a past history of obstetric vasculopathies are those in whom preventive measures can help.

As per the National Institute for Health and Care Excellence (NICE) guidelines, women are at an increased risk of pre-eclampsia if they have one high-risk factor or more than one moderate-risk factor for pre-eclampsia.[3]

The high-risk factors include:

- Hypertensive disease in a previous pregnancy,
- Chronic kidney disease,
- Autoimmune disease, such as systemic lupus erythematosus (SLE) or antiphospholipid antibody (APA) syndrome,
- Type 1 or type 2 diabetes and
- Chronic hypertension.

Moderate risk factors include:

- First pregnancy,
- Age ≤40 years,
- Pregnancy interval ≤10 years,
- Body mass index (BMI) ≤35 kg/m^2 at first visit,
- Family history of pre-eclampsia and
- Multiple pregnancy.

SALT RESTRICTION

In a society like ours where food and rest are given undue importance in day-to-day life for well-being and health, a low-salt diet or even a salt-free diet is suggested more often than not by the pregnant woman and her family, rather than the attending obstetrician, for preventing pre-eclampsia. When the doctor announces that the pregnant woman tends to develop a rise in blood pressure, the first response is a salt-free diet. Worse still is a situation when the doctor is informed on subsequent visits that the family has stopped serving the pregnant woman food containing salt! All this when the medical staff has never advised such a step.

Although high blood pressure before pregnancy is associated with a risk of gestational hypertension and pre-eclampsia, no convincing evidence has been produced to show that dietary salt reduction helps in the prevention and treatment of hypertension during pregnancy. Thus, current guidelines do not recommend a sodium restriction during pregnancy to prevent gestational hypertension and the development of pre-eclampsia.[4]

It seems that the concept of a salt-free diet is deeply ingrained in society for the prevention of hypertension. This thinking comes from experiences of elderly subjects in the family who are having age-related hypertension and have been advised to consume a low salt or salt-free diet by their attending physician and a quick and hasty extrapolation is done. Little do they realize that both are different conditions, and hypertension is the only external manifestation common to both. Although it is well-known that salt-free or low salt diets do not in any way help in managing or preventing hypertensive disorders of pregnancy, in fact, the results might be reversed. It is well possible that in an overzealous attempt to restrict salt in the mother, the foetus suffers from vital electrolyte deprivation. There is some fear that maternal salt restriction may produce stunting of foetal growth.

A piece of popular advice given by obstetricians of the Indian subcontinent is to avoid consuming salt-rich foods, for example, pickles. However, this has not been scientifically validated and therefore, seems to be advice given by convention or by the word of mouth. It has not been proved to give any great advantage to the woman who is hypertensive or potentially hypertensive.

DIURETICS

The use of diuretics for preventing pre-eclampsia is a habit that obstetricians seem to have borrowed from their physician counterparts. This habit seems to be more confined to the senior generation of obstetric practitioners because probably the youngest of the lot seem to be aware that these do not help in preventing pre-eclampsia but also may, in fact, cause complications. The use of these agents is also instituted in subjects with oedema in pre-eclampsia.

One small African study examined the effect of furosemide on hypertension and oedema in patients with pre-eclampsia experiencing high cardiac output. These were all women with late-onset pre-eclampsia. The study enrolled only 14 patients. Lower cardiac output, systolic blood pressure and diastolic blood pressure were recorded after furosemide administration with patient heart rates remaining stable. This encouraged the authors to conclude that the stability of the heart rate suggested that the change of cardiac output was as a result of a decrease in blood volume. They suggested that diuretics could be useful in the management of late-onset pre-eclampsia, indicating that an increase in water retention could play a role in the development of late-onset pre-eclampsia.[5] However, too small a sample size eliminates the use of this study in clinical practice.

For one who knows the pathophysiology of oedema in pre-eclampsia well, it is not difficult to guess the error in this decision of prescribing a diuretic for treating oedema of pre-eclampsia. Oedema in pre-eclampsia is not a result of an increase in the circulating fluid load. In pre-eclampsia, oedema occurs because of altered albumin distribution as well as the loosening of the vascular wall cellular arrangements. Therefore, using diuretics to treat oedema of pre-eclampsia or prevent pre-eclampsia occurrence is both irrational and even harmful. It is feared that long-term use of diuretics in pregnant women can in fact lead to worsening of IUGR. This seems to be the result of the drastic electrolyte loss that occurs in the process of diuresis. Therefore, the use of diuretics in the prevention of pre-eclampsia or treatment of oedema in women with pre-eclampsia is only mentioned to be condemned.

ANTIHYPERTENSIVES

The uses of antihypertensives have been proposed by some for subjects of chronic hypertension. In these women, continuing the use of antihypertensives on which she has been stabilised is in order. However, expecting this antihypertensive to prevent the superimposition of pre-eclampsia over the under running chronic hypertension may not work. Chronic hypertension may be controlled, but in no way is the occurrence of pre-eclampsia prevented. Two critical analyses have also corroborated this contention.[6]

CALCIUM SUPPLEMENTATION

Dietary calcium and extraneous calcium supplementation to specifically prevent pre-eclampsia caught the attention of obstetric scientists. Fodor et al. reviewed this matter in detail. They felt that calcium supplementation seems to be a good opportunity to prevent pre-eclampsia.[7] One more study that initiated the thought process in this regard was performed by Belizean et al. In this study, an inverse association was found between dietary calcium intake and the development of pre-eclampsia. It, therefore, meant that if the calcium content of the diet was low then there was a higher chance for the woman to develop pre-eclampsia.[8] These two studies invited a series of activities for calcium supplement for reducing the incidence of pre-eclampsia.

Though most of the world started agreeing, they missed one vital concept. In countries like India, calcium supplementation for pregnant women has been a routine for decades. It would have been pertinent to study the behaviour of pre-eclampsia in these societies. However, based on these types of publications cited, a series of studies got published in many journals. Most of these studies extolled the virtue of calcium supplementation during pregnancy for preventing pre-eclampsia. However, as usually happens in modern medicine, all studies were not so positive about this. This initiated an undertaking of a large review of all such published data at the Cochrane Database. This review tries to find some answers to the questions: Does calcium supplementation prevent pre-eclampsia? If the answer to the first was yes, then in what dose? A meta-analysis of a large number of studies on this matter showed calcium supplementation appears to almost halve the risk of pre-eclampsia and to reduce the rare occurrence of the composite outcome "death or serious morbidity". There were no other clear benefits or harms.[8] But this had a rider attached to it: Calcium supplementation would help only those women in whom dietary intake of calcium was already low and would effectively reduce pre-eclampsia.

In 2015, a meta-analysis and systematic review emerged that seriously shook the applecart of calcium supplementation in the prevention of pre-eclampsia.[9] Results of this study found that though calcium supplementation reduced the overall risk of pre-eclampsia in 10 trials, its effect was larger in two subgroups: Low-baseline calcium intake and increased risk of developing hypertensive disorders. This effect was not significant amongst larger studies. It concluded that some evidence for calcium supplementation exists, but its use is limited by the possibility of publication bias and a lack of large trials. Currently, the focus is on calcium and vitamin D supplementation for the prevention of pre-eclampsia.

OTHER TRACE ELEMENTS AND MICRONUTRIENTS

The possibility of magnesium in preventing pre-eclampsia got examined because magnesium sulphate is used successfully in eclampsia and severe pre-eclampsia to prevent convulsions. Obstetric scientists wanted to explore if it was effective at preventing pre-eclampsia altogether. Magnesium supplementation through diet or tablets containing magnesium failed to produce any significant change in the causation of pre-eclampsia.[10,11]

Similarly, zinc supplementation in pregnancy does not influence the course of pre-eclampsia in any way worth mentioning. Though levels of zinc in plasma and the leucocytes may be reduced in pre-eclampsia, counteracting this by extraneous zinc supplementation seems to be simple and irrational. Despite positive clinical and in vitro data, strong evidence to support periconceptional supplementation of other micronutrients for reducing the risk of pre-eclampsia is still lacking. Further studies are also needed to evaluate the benefit of nutritional supplementation such as chocolate and long-chain polyunsaturated fatty acids.[12]

ASPIRIN FOR THE PREVENTION OF PRE-ECLAMPSIA

Aspirin is maximally researched and used in the prevention of obstetric vasculopathies including pre-eclampsia. Large meta-analyses including antiplatelet agents, largely low-dose aspirin, have moderate benefits when used for prevention of pre-eclampsia and its consequences.[13] In this section, the role of aspirin in the prevention of pre-eclampsia is examined.

POSSIBLE MECHANISM OF ACTION OF ASPIRIN

Obstetric vasculopathies including pre-eclampsia have vasospasm as their basic pathology. It is during this vasospasm that blood circulation slows down. During this sluggish phase of blood circulation, the lipids, low-density lipoprotein (LDL) and very-low-density lipoprotein (VLDL) tend to go closer to the activated endothelial lining. Some sink into the intercellular spaces. This is the space between two endothelial cells. In the intercellular space, the free radicals are on the prowl. They quickly denature the lipid (VLDL and LDL) molecules that have sunk within. These free radicals have been generated by the activated endothelial lining at the foetomaternal interface. The endothelial activation has the failure of trophoblastic invasion and inefficient spiral arteriolar moulding at its root. This matter has been extensively discussed in chapters related to aetiopathology of pre-eclampsia.

Once denatured by the free radicals, the lipid molecules get flushed into the system when vasospasm is reduced and reperfusion results. In the phase of reperfusion, the denatured lipids go into the circulation. Wherever they go, the denatured lipid molecules produce vasospasm. It generates a vicious cycle of vasospasm – reperfusion – vasospasm. When it involves the entire maternal vasculature, it results in pre-eclampsia.

Aspirin does not release the vasospasm. It acts by preventing the sluggishness of bloodstream while facing the obstruction of reduced vessel calibre in vasospasm. It tends to act by keeping the blood "more liquid" (words used in common parlance). As a result, the blood continues to flow, and the VLDLs and LDLs find it extremely difficult to come close to the endothelial lining. Resultantly, these lipids do not have enough time to sink into the intercellular spaces. It prevents denaturation and subsequent reperfusion damage. A sluggish bloodstream is a strong prerequisite for the entire pathophysiology of pre-eclampsia to get triggered. Aspirin treats the effect of sluggishness and not the cause (vasospasm and reperfusion damages).

Studies that have concentrated on the dominant effect of aspirin on thromboxane-prostacyclin imbalance in the prevention of pre-eclampsia have therefore produced inconsistent results. Those that concentrate on the balance expect aspirin to combat the cause of pre-eclampsia. Aspirin, on the contrary, is preventing the effects and not the cause. It prevents the sluggishness of bloodstream. If the cause is intact and the effect is combated, then the results are bound to be inconsistent. By whatever means, if the cause is neutralised, the efficacy would be most consistent. Aspirin, therefore, has disillusioned those who concentrated on it as the treatment of the cause. On the other hand, those who have grasped the entire pathophysiology in greater depth of both the disease as well as treating agents are not surprised by the lack of universal consistency in results of aspirin.

ASPIRIN: REVIEW OF LITERATURE

Having had examined and discussed the intricacies of aspirin in the prevention of pre-eclampsia, it will be worthwhile to review the literature published on this matter. The obstetric world started using low-dose aspirin long before big reviews and meta-analysis started appearing in research publications. Small studies and convincing results in clinical practice seemed to have led the success story. Large reviews came much later. So hesitant and shy to accept the efficacy of aspirin, it took decades after which researchers and reviewers accepted that aspirin was indeed effective in preventing pre-eclampsia.

Two large multicentre trials were undertaken, popularly known as CLASP and ECPPA trials.[14,15] These studies too were typically hesitant in concluding the effectiveness of aspirin. They qualified that only proteinuric pre-eclampsia gets prevented convincingly with aspirin. They showed "limited utility" of low-dose aspirin in the prevention of pre-eclampsia. The CLASP study did show a reduction in the incidence of proteinuric hypertension and IUGR. However, these and other large trials were roundly criticized for poor compliance, gestational age at randomisation and heterogeneity of dosage of the drug, etc. Despite this, doubts were raised about the efficacy of aspirin in consistently reducing the incidence of pre-eclampsia.

An example of a hesitant review could be traced in 2007.[13] The reviewers' state that overall the administration of antiplatelet agents to women at risk leads to a 17% reduction in the risk of developing pre-eclampsia. Amongst women in the primary prevention trials, for every 72 women treated, 1 case of pre-eclampsia was prevented. However, for high-risk women, only 19 need to be treated to prevent 1 case. There are also smaller reductions in the risk of preterm birth (8%) and of foetal or neonatal death (14%), with larger numbers of women needed to be treated to prevent such outcomes. Overall, adverse effects appear to be low but underreporting makes it difficult to be confident about this, especially where higher doses are used. As most of the evidence relates to low-dose aspirin, this is the antiplatelet agent that should be used in clinical practice for the prevention of pre-eclampsia. Starting aspirin before 12 weeks or using higher doses, or both, cannot be recommended for clinical practice until more information is available about the safety of these approaches.[13]

One study performed a meta-analysis to assess the influence of gestational age at the time of introduction of low-dose aspirin on the incidence of pre-eclampsia in women at increased risk based on abnormal uterine artery Doppler. It was found that low-dose aspirin treatment initiated early in pregnancy is an efficient method of reducing the incidence of pre-eclampsia and its consequences in women with ultrasonographic evidence of abnormal placentation diagnosed by uterine artery Doppler studies.[16] A series of studies on this matter was subjected to a meta-analysis that concluded that aspirin in low-dose is highly effective in preventing obstetric vasculopathies, especially pre-eclampsia and IUGR.[17]

WHAT DOSE OF ASPIRIN: 75 MG OR 150 MG?

Traditionally, aspirin is used in a dose of 300–500 mg/day for uses other than for the prevention of pre-eclampsia. But for prevention of obstetric vasculopathies including pre-eclampsia, this dose is not found to be necessary and can be downright harmful. The recommended dose of aspirin for this indication, therefore, is 1.2 mg/kg/day. This will come to 75–150 mg/day in an average-sized woman.

As early as in 1988, our group started studying and publishing our results on pre-eclampsia remote from term.[18] Since then we have been consistently getting good results with low-dose aspirin used in a dose of 1.2 mg/kg of body weight of the pregnant woman. This on an average came to 75 mg/day in Indian women from whom all our data was generated and published.[19,20] After these initial publications, we went on regularly documenting and publishing our results on different obstetric vasculopathies, including pre-eclampsia remote from term.[21–25] We have been using this dose since then and have not found it necessary to give higher doses.

It was in 2017 that a paper was published, which studied the use of the Fetal Medicine Foundation (FMF) algorithm in clinical practice. It was called the Aspirin for Evidence-Based PREeclampsia Prevention (ASPRE) trial.[26] This trial was designed to propose aspirin as a treatment for primary prevention of pre-eclampsia in all patients considered to be at high risk following first-trimester combined screening. This multicentre, double-blind, randomised, placebo-controlled trial evaluated the effect of prophylactic low-dose aspirin administered in the first trimester of pregnancy on the incidence of delivery with pre-eclampsia before 37 weeks of gestation in patients at high risk. Patients considered at high risk were randomised to either a group that was given aspirin (150 mg/day, taken at bedtime) or a group given a placebo. Treatment was started in the first trimester (between 11 and 14 weeks of gestation) and continued to 36 weeks of gestation. In this study, the dose of 150 mg/day was selected based on previous evidence of a dose-dependent benefit. This study showed good prevention efficacy with aspirin in a dose of 150 mg.[27] Aspirin efficacy for the prevention of pre-eclampsia is dose-dependent, but the optimum dosage, 75 mg/day to 150 mg/day, needs to be determined. Safety data at 150 mg/day are still limited. Until a time as this issue is settled, one need not change the policy that is being practiced by clinicians currently in their clinical practices. This means that those clinicians who are still prescribing 75 mg can continue to do so. However, if one has already switched to 150 mg then that should be continued. There is no need to change the policy until final word on safety of larger dose of aspirin is published.

MISGIVINGS AND FEARS ABOUT ASPIRIN

There were two principal fears about aspirin: First, the possibility of haemorrhage if a pregnant woman needs any operative intervention, including caesarean section when she is on aspirin, and second, the possibility of premature closure of ductus arteriosus because of the use of aspirin – a nonsteroidal anti-inflammatory drug (NSAID). Both these fears were subsequently allayed. The understanding of COX-1 and COX-2 receptors and the role of COX-2 receptors in maintaining the patency of the ductus during intra-uterine life was of great significance. Aspirin and other NSAIDs act on COX-1 receptors. Thus, they do not come in the way of patency of ductus arteriosus.

The second fear was based on the fact that aspirin acts by permanently paralysing the platelets. Any surgeon would be scared of the possibility of operating on a subject with an ongoing aspirin regimen. The solution, however, lies in the fact that in obstetrics low-dose aspirin are used. This will not have as much an extensive effect on the platelets as would a regular dose of aspirin (300 mgm). The effects of aspirin are dose-dependent.[28] As a result, even if operative intervention is required, the field may get a little more sanguine. But the bleeding is never profuse. Any reasonably experienced obstetrician can easily handle this platelet ooze by taking tight stitches.

ASPIRIN TIMING

Recent research publications have shown that administering aspirin at night before bed is most effective. Aspirin given during other times during the day is not that effective.[26] Many clinicians have recently switched over to this time of the day for administering aspirin.

REFERENCES

1. Desai P: *Obstetric Vasculopathies: Delhi*, 2013, New Delhi, Jaypee Publishers.
2. Lindheimer M, Roberts J, Cunningham F, Chesley L: In Lindheimer M, Roberts J, and Cunningham F, editors: *Chesley, Hypertensive Disorders of Pregnancy*, 2nd ed., p. 36, 1998, Stamford, Appleton & Lange.

3. National Institute for Health and Care Excellence (NICE) NICE CG 107: *Hypertension in Pregnancy: The Management of Hypertensive Disorders During Pregnancy*, 2010, Manchester, UK: National Institute for Health and Clinical Excellence. [Accessed February 5, 2015]. Available from www.nice.org.uk/guidance/cg107/resources/guidance-hypertension-in-pregnancy-pdf.

4. Asayama K, Imai Y. The impact of salt intake during and after pregnancy. *Hypertens Res* 41(1):1–5, 2018. doi:10.1038/hr.2017.90.

5. Tamás P, Hantosi E, Farkas B, Ifi Z, Betlehem J, Bódis J: Preliminary study of the effects of furosemide on blood pressure during late-onset pre-eclampsia in patients with high cardiac output. *Int J Gynaecol Obstet* 136(1):87–90, 2017. doi:10.1002/ijgo.12019.

6. Sibai B: Treatment of hypertension in pregnancy women. *N Engl J Med* 335: 257–265, 1996.

7. Fodor A, Gyorffy A, Váradi M, Fülesdi B, Major T: The possible options for the prevention of preeclampsia. *Orv Hetil* 153(4):144–151, 2012.

8. Belizean J, Villar J, Repke J: The relationship between calcium intake and pregnancy induced hypertension: Up-to-date evidence. *Am J Obstet. Gynecol* 158: 898–902, 1988.

9. Tang R, Tang IC, Henry A, Welsh A: Limited evidence for calcium supplementation in preeclampsia prevention: A meta-analysis and systematic review. *Hypertens Pregnancy* 34(2):181–203, 2015. doi: 10.3109/10641955.2014.988353.

10. Briceño-Pérez C, Briceño-Sanabria L, Vigil-De Gracia P: Prediction and prevention of preeclampsia. *Hypertens Pregnancy* 28(2):138–155, 2009.

11. Oken E, Ning Y, Rifas-Shiman S, Rich-Edwards J, Olsen S, Gillman M: Diet during pregnancy and risk of preeclampsia or gestational hypertension. *Ann Epidemiol* 17(9):663–668, 2007.

12. Achamrah N, Ditisheim A: Nutritional approach to preeclampsia prevention. *Curr Opin Clin Nutr Metab Care* 21(3):168–173, 2018. doi:10.1097/MCO.0000000000000462.

13. Duley L, Henderson-Smart DJ, Meher S, King JF: Antiplatelet agents for preventing pre-eclampsia and its complications. *Cochrane Database Syst Rev* (2), Art. No.: CD004659, 2007. doi:10.1002/14651858.CD004659.pub2.

14. CLASP: A randomized trial of low dose aspirin in prevention and treatment of pre-eclampsia among 9364 pregnant women. *Lancet* 343:619–629, 1994.

15. ECPPA: Randomized trial of low dose aspirin for the prevention of maternal and fetal complications' in high-risk pregnant women. *Br J Obstet Gynecol* 103:39–47, 1996.

16. Bujold E, Morency A, Roberge S, Lacasse Y, Forest J, Giguère Y: Acetylsalicylic acid for the prevention of preeclampsia and intra-uterine growth restriction in women with abnormal uterine artery Doppler: A systematic review and meta-analysis. *J Obstet Gynaecol Can* 31(9):818–826, 2009.

17. Bujold E, Roberge S, Lacasse Y, Bureau M, Audibert F, Marcoux S, Forest J, Giguère Y: Prevention of preeclampsia and intrauterine growth restriction with aspirin started in early pregnancy: A meta-analysis. *Obstet Gynecol* 116(2 Pt 1):402–414, 2010.

18. Desai P, Chandrasekhar G, Udvani HH, Hazra M: Preeclampsia of early onset. *J Obstet Gynaecol India* 38(5):548, 1988.

19. Bharadwaj R, Desai M, Desai P: Low dose aspirin in prevention of IUGR: A double blind prospective randomized case controlled study. *J Obstet Gynaecol India* 45(4):445–448, 1994.

20. Desai P, Rao S: Role of low dose aspirin in mothers registering high serum HCG levels at mid trimester. *J Obstet Gynaecol India* 52(5):30–32, 2002.

21. Desai P, Desai M, Modi D: Preeclampsia of early onset: Recurrence risks and long term effects. *J Obstet Gynaecol India* 44(6):855–859, 1994.

22. Desai P: Pre-eclampsia remote from term and A. P. A. syndrome: Examining the association. *J Obstet Gynaecol India* 47:484, 1997.

23. Desai P, Anand R: APA syndrome and recurrent missed abortions and stillbirths. *J Obstet Gynaecol India* 48(7):28, 1998.

24. Desai P, Anand RS, Desai M, Modi D: Effect of treatment on cases testing positive for APA: A prospective study. *J Obstet Gynaecol India* 50(2):34–36, 2000.

25. Desai P, Shah A: Longitudinal observations of deterioration of CTG parameters in subjects with adverse outcomes of APA syndrome. *J Obstet Gynaecol India* 53(3):244–247, 2003.

26. Rolnik DL, Wright D, Poon LC, O'Gorman N, Syngelaki A, de Paco Matallana C, Akolekar R et al: Aspirin versus placebo in pregnancies at high risk for preterm preeclampsia. *N Engl J Med* 377(7):613–622, 2017.

27. Roberge S, Nicolaides K, Demers S, Hyett J, Chaillet N, Bujold E: The role of aspirin dose on the prevention of preeclampsia and fetal growth restriction: Systematic review and meta-analysis. *Am J Obstet Gynecol* 216(2):110–120.e6, 2017.

28. Atallah A, Lecarpentier E, Goffinet F, Doret-Dion M, Gaucherand P, Tsatsaris V: Aspirin for prevention of preeclampsia. *Drugs* 77(17):1819–1831, 2017.

PART 5

Systemic manifestations

9

Central nervous system

CHANGES IN THE CNS

CNS involvement in pre-eclampsia seems to be occurring more regularly then that borne by clinical findings. Also, it increases as the condition worsens from mild pre-eclampsia to severe pre-eclampsia and eclampsia. Abnormal cranial MRI findings were reported in 6% of women with pre-eclampsia, in 36% of women with severe pre-eclampsia, and in 92% of women with eclampsia.[1]

The clinical manifestations (plural) of CNS involvement may appear quite late in the disease progression. In one study, a non-invasive diffusion-weighted MRI technique, intravoxel incoherent motion, was used to study cerebral perfusion on the capillary level and cerebral oedema in women with pre-eclampsia, normal pregnancy and non-pregnant women. It was found that the cerebral perfusion measures were comparable between the study groups, except for a portion of the basal ganglia where hypoperfusion was detected in pre-eclampsia but not in a normal pregnancy or non-pregnant women.[2] In some pregnant women, however, the CNS may get affected more readily.

The preference given to the CNS by the human body can also be seen in the foetus. In states of chronic hypoxia like intrauterine growth restriction (IUGR) and pre-eclampsia, oxygenation of the foetal brain is affected late and more likely as a terminal event. This is a well-observed phenomenon on colour Doppler studies where the foetal circulation gets adjusted to hypoxia and the foetal CNS oxygenation is maintained until the end. Once foetal CNS oxygenation gets affected, terminal eventualities follow if quick intervention is not done.

It has been found that women who report headache in severe pre-eclampsia just before having an eclamptic convulsion have abnormal cerebral perfusion. This was shown through colour Doppler studies.[3] Abnormal cerebral perfusion is a result of vasospasm.

The most dreaded clinical feature of CNS changes of pre-eclampsia is its stage of convulsions known as eclampsia. If a subject progresses to eclampsia, it shows that apparently the pre-eclampsia may have been neglected. Rarely, some subjects have an increased susceptibility to CNS manifestations. In those women, eclampsia occurs much more quickly once pre-eclampsia is registered clinically. Interestingly a familial tendency to the development of eclampsia, in women with preeclampsia has also been reported.[4]

PATHOLOGICAL LESIONS IN PRE-ECLAMPSIA

The classical description of pathological features of CNS changes in pre-eclampsia includes ischaemic lesions, oedema and perivascular micro-haemorrhage.[5] These changes are characteristic of vasospasm and subsequent reperfusion damage that occurs in pre-eclampsia. Extensive documentation of CNS changes in pre-eclampsia and eclampsia has been done by Sheehan and Lynch.[6] They showed 76 types of lesions in 48 subjects on post-mortem who died of eclampsia. Of these, the most common were piaarachnoid haemorrhages, cortical petechiae, subcortical petechiae and multiple small focal softening or petechiae in the white matter or midbrain. Their accounts are excellently detailed, and they brilliantly fit into one common explanation reperfusion damage of obstetric vasculopathies, including pre-eclampsia. Many others have documented these or similar changes in women with severe preeclampsia or eclampsia who were alive. However, their descriptions just complete the list without adding significantly to the understanding of the pathological process.

Brain

On gross examination, oedema is found post-convulsion, which means that cerebral oedema is not the cause of convulsions but the effect of the same. Administration of mannitol may reduce this oedema. However, mannitol can produce severe complications like pulmonary oedema and volume overload in a strained cardiovascular system of women with eclampsia. This could even prove fatal. Therefore, it is no longer used in modern obstetrics.

As regards those capillaries that did not break, they show evidence of stasis of circulation. This was indicated by fibrin deposition. Once again, this is a manifestation of vasospasm. It is possible that this stasis may not be confined to the capillaries but also to the pre-capillary segments of vessels wherein too this type of fibrin deposition may extend. Stasis following vasospasm and then after reperfusion damage produces fibrin deposition near the petechial haemorrhages.

POSTERIOR LEUKOENCEPHALOPATHY SYNDROME

Posterior leukoencephalopathy syndrome is a relatively recently documented brain disorder in pre-eclampsia and eclampsia. It predominantly affects the cerebral white matter. This syndrome is characterised by neuroimaging findings of reversible vasogenic subcortical oedema without infarction.[7] Oedematous lesions particularly involve the posterior parietal and occipital lobes and may spread to basal ganglia, brainstem and cerebellum.[8] On MRI, the lesions typically show diffuse areas of increased intensity, which selectively involves the parieto-occipital white matter. It is a fast-progressing condition that is clinically characterised by nausea and vomiting, headache, visual disturbances, altered sensorium, convulsions and occasionally, focal neurological insufficiency. Posterior leuko-encephalopathy syndrome is often associated with

an abrupt increase in blood pressure and is usually seen in patients with eclampsia, renal disease and hypertensive encephalopathy.[8] Early recognition of this condition is of paramount importance because prompt control of blood pressure can stem its progression. Delay in the diagnosis and treatment can result in permanent damage to affected brain tissues.

PSYCHIATRIC COMPLICATIONS FOLLOWING OBSTETRIC VASCULOPATHIES: ANY CORRELATION?

In 2004, some animal studies hinted that exposure to hypertensive disorders in pregnancy may be associated with an increased risk for later development of schizophrenia.[9] However, the latest study that pooled data included 23 studies and 15 studies found that hypertensive disorders of pregnancy had a negative impact for at least one mental or behavioural disorder. The pooled effect of 11 studies included in the meta-analysis showed that pre-eclampsia was associated with increased risk of offspring schizophrenia. The authors were, therefore, inconclusive on the effect of hypertensive disorders of pregnancy and other mental and behavioural disorders. They suggested further high-quality, large sample, and birth cohort studies are needed to further progress this area of research.[10]

REFERENCES

1. Osmanağaoğlu MA, Dinç G, Osmanağaoğlu S, Dinç H, Bozkaya H: Comparison of cerebral magnetic resonance and electro-encephalogram findings in pre-eclamptic and eclamptic women. *Aust N Z J Obstet Gynaecol* 45(5):384–390, 2005.
2. Nelander M, Hannsberger D, Sundström-Poromaa I, Bergman L, Weis J, Åkerud H, Wikström J, Wikström AK. Assessment of cerebral perfusion and edema in preeclampsia with intravoxel incoherent motion MRI. *Acta Obstet Gynecol Scand* 97(10):1212–1218, 2018. doi:10.1111/aogs.13383. Epub 2018 Jun 12.

3. Dusse LM, Alpoim PN, Silva JT, Rios DR, Brandão AH, Cabral AC: Revisiting HELLP syndrome. *Clin Chim Acta* 451(Pt B):117–120. doi:10.1016/j.cca.2015.10.024. Epub 2015 Oct 23.

4. Sibbai B, Spinnato J, Watson D: Eclampsia IV. Neurological findings and future outcome. *Am J Obstet Gynecol* 152:184–192, 1985.

5. Topuz S, Kalelioğlu I, Iyibozkurt A, Akhan S, Has R, Tunaci M, Ibrahimoğlu L: Cranial imaging spectrum in hypertensive disease of pregnancy. *Clin Exp Obstet Gynecol* 35(3):194–197, 2008.

6. Sheehan H, Lynch J: Cerebral lesions. In: Sheehan H, Lynch J editors: *Pathology of Toxemia of Pregnancy*, Chapter 32. pp. 524–553, 1973, Baltimore, MD, Williams & Wilkins.

7. Lee VH, Wijdicks EFM, Manno EM, Rabinstein AA: Clinical spectrum of reversible posterior leukoencephalopathy syndrome. *Arch Neurol* 65(2):205–210, 2008. doi:10.1001/archneurol.2007.46.

8. Garg RK: Posterior leukoencephalopathy syndrome. *Postgrad Med J* 77(903):24–28, 2001.

9. Boksa P: Animal models of obstetric complications in relation to schizophrenia. *Brain Res Rev* 45(1):1–17, 2004.

10. Dachew BA, Mamun A, Maravilla JC, Alati R: Association between hypertensive disorders of pregnancy and the development of offspring mental and behavioural problems: A systematic review and meta-analysis. *Psychiatry Res* 260:458–467, 2018. doi:10.1016/j.psychres.2017.12.027.

10

Cardiovascular system

CHANGES IN CARDIAC FUNCTIONS

Physiological changes in cardiac function occur early in pregnancy. This may be as early as the luteal phase of the menstrual cycle.[1] Savu et al. assessed the performance of the left ventricle (LV) in normal, uncomplicated pregnancies while considering the actual left ventricular load and shape. Cardiac output increased during pregnancy because of a higher stroke volume early in pregnancy and a late increase in heart rate, whereas the total vascular resistance decreased. The progressive development of eccentric hypertrophy was observed, which subsequently recovered postpartum. Sphericity index (SI) decreased physiologically from the first to the third trimesters and returned postpartum to values comparable to the control. The SI is used to evaluate the shape of the right and left ventricles of the heart and is derived by calculating the ratio between the end-diastolic mid-basal-apical and transverse lengths. Although higher ventricular stroke work was noted toward the third trimester, ejection fraction showed no significant changes.[2] It seems the SI does not get affected by pre-eclampsia. No good published data is available specifically on this aspect of pre-eclampsia.

STROKE VOLUME AND HEART RATE

Cardiac output is calculated as cardiac rate is multiplied by stroke volume. So, a rise in cardiac output could be the result of a rise in either one or both. The increase in cardiac output is a function of the rise in heart rate until about 32 weeks of pregnancy. Similarly, the volume of blood emitted at every heartbeat expressed as stroke volume increases early in pregnancy. It steadies by 15 weeks of pregnancy. Both these rises get reflected in the rise in cardiac output during pregnancy.

HOW DOES THE HEART INCREASE ITS CARDIAC OUTPUT?

It is not difficult to understand this complex phenomenon. The cardiac muscle acts as a pump. An increase in cardiac output means the pump needs

1. Extra fluid to push,
2. To increase its pumping capacity, and
3. An unhindered outflow system.

All the three in combination will increase the output. This is shown clearly in Figure 10.1. As a result, the amount of blood that reaches the target organs and tissues in pregnancy increases.

Increase in the fluid supplied to the heart is ensured by the increase in preload. In a healthy pregnancy, this preload is efficiently pumped out through a robust cardiac musculature. The final step of smooth and unhindered outflow is ensured by the reduced peripheral resistance in normal pregnancy.

As regards the pumping efficiency of cardiac musculature, all three components that can contribute to better pumping are increased. The thickness of cardiac musculature, the size of the cardiac chambers, and the contractile power of the cardiac muscle mass and size leads to an increased amount of blood being competently pushed out. A small but significant contribution to this comes from the increase in heart rate. All of these together combine as a team effort to bring about an increase in cardiac output in pregnancy.

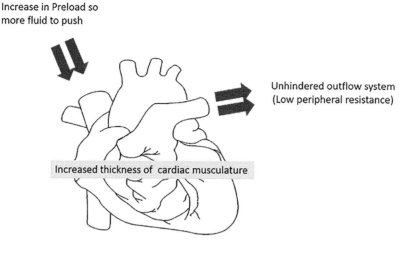

Increase in Preload so
more fluid to push

Unhindered outflow system
(Low peripheral resistance)

Increased thickness of cardiac musculature

How Does Cardiac Output Increase In Pregnancy

Figure 10.1 Increase in cardiac output.

VASCULAR RESPONSE TO INCREASE CARDIAC OUTPUT

The amount of blood in circulation and the amount of blood pushed out by the heart are both increased in normal pregnancy. To accommodate this increase in the volume of blood forced out by the heart, the vascular channels through which the blood circulates gets more accommodative. This is done by the second wave of trophoblastic invasion. The second wave of trophoblastic invasion converts the vascular channels at the voluminous foetomaternal interface to a low-resistance pool. Consequently, the blood volume meets less resistance and flows easily.

Nevertheless, changes in vascular modelling occur relatively late in pregnancy. On the other hand, the changes like those in blood volume take place much earlier. As a result, the body makes some changes early in pregnancy. One of these changes is the in oscillatory pressure along the vessels lining. This is an interesting phenomenon.

OSCILLATORY PRESSURE AND PROPULSIVE PRESSURE

When the blood mass pumped out with great force from the heart strikes the vessel wall, the vessel wall has two types of pressures to bear.

One pressure is generated along the vessel wall which does not have any propulsive function. It is the oscillatory pressure. It gets distributed along the vascular lining. It is like the force lashing waves generates on the rocks along the seashore. The other pressure is propulsive. It is that force of blood which is excess of the oscillatory pressure and drives the blood along the vessel wall. It can be measured as total pressure on the vessel wall minus the oscillatory pressure. This pressure is functionally important. It is influenced by the pulsatility of the vessel wall and therefore, plays an important role in facilitating the increase in blood volume and power of flow during pregnancy. This is shown explicitly in Figure 10.2.

Because of increased pulsatility of vessel walls, the oscillatory pressure is effectively combated. The vessel walls can withstand the force of the lashing of blood effectively in normal pregnancy. The component of increased pulsatility which is not used in resisting the onslaught of oscillatory pressure is used to propel the blood forward. Increased pulsatility of the vessel wall, therefore, accommodates the increased blood volume being pushed out of the heart of the pregnant woman efficiently. This occurs early in pregnancy.

In pre-eclampsia, there is an interesting breakdown of the accommodative mechanism. Initially, the flexible vessels accommodate the

Oscillatory and Propulsive pressures

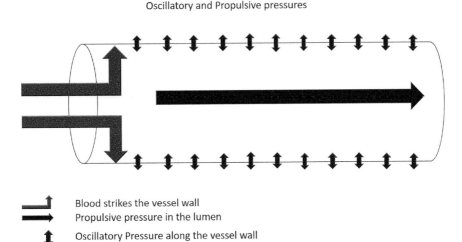

Blood strikes the vessel wall
Propulsive pressure in the lumen

Oscillatory Pressure along the vessel wall

Figure 10.2 Oscillatory and propulsive pressures.

increased oscillatory pressure. The progressive rise in blood pressure that occurs in preeclampsia causes the blood to flow with much greater pressure. The vessels, especially the arteries, respond by further increasing their pulsatility. As a result, they allow the non-propulsive force to efficiently distribute along the vessel wall without breaking the wall. Also, the propulsive component of these vessels is increased, whereby the blood can flow through a narrowed vessel lumen without much problem. However, the power of accommodation of the vessels is not limitless. At some unpredictable stage, the vessel wall can give way. This is seen in accidental haemorrhage, intracranial haemorrhage in severe pre-eclampsia and subcapsular haemorrhage in the liver. Also, the deposition of fibrin complexes along the vessel walls as seen in preeclampsia reduces the flexibility. As a result, the vessel walls become vulnerable to rupture.

PERIPHERAL VASCULAR RESISTANCE

The body of the gravida makes all possible arrangements to ensure smooth and unobstructed blood flow to the critical organs of her body, including the uterus. Reduction in peripheral resistance is one step in this direction. Peripheral resistance seems to be most vulnerable to a pathological onslaught of pre-eclampsia.

A rise in peripheral resistance resulting from different complementary processes makes the maternal system sense the challenge faced by the circulating bloodstream. If the maternal system has a high peripheral resistance, maternal systems raise a woman's blood pressure which clinically manifests as pre-eclampsia. In a study published in 2012, it was found that during normal pregnancy there is an increase in cardiac output and decrease in blood pressure and peripheral arterial resistance, whereas central aortic properties are less altered.[2]

CHANGES IN VENOUS SYSTEM

Simultaneously as the arterial and other components of the cardiovascular system undergo a series of changes in normal pregnancy as well as in pre-eclampsia, the venous musculature and tone also adjust to these changes. The venous walls seem to be passively accommodative. In the absence of a muscular resistance, the venous vessels can dilate passively without a need for large adjustments. Thus, the passive accommodations by venous system assisted by strong skeletal muscle activity that surround these venous lining (e.g., gastrocnemius muscles) propel the increased venous circulation towards the heart in pregnancy. The venous system, therefore, undergoes changes which can best be described as limited.

REFERENCES

1. Spaanderman M, Van Beek E, Ekhart T, Van Eyck J, Cheriex E, De Leeuw P, Peeters L: Changes in hemodynamic parameters and volume homeostasis with the menstrual cycle among women with a history of preeclampsia. *Am J Obstet Gynecol* 182(5):1127–1134, 2000.

2. Savu O, Jurcuţ R, Giuşcă S, van Mieghem T, Gussi I, Popescu B, Ginghină C, Rademakers F, Deprest J, Voigt J: Morphological and functional adaptation of the maternal heart during pregnancy. *Circ Cardiovasc Imaging* 5(3):289–297, 2012.

11

Haematological system

INTRODUCTION

Numerous haematological changes have been found in pre-eclampsia. The commonest and most consistent is the development of thrombocytopenia. Thrombocytopenia can occur in many medical syndromes complicating pregnancy. These include pre-eclampsia and severe pre-eclampsia complicated by haemolysis with elevated liver enzymes and low platelets (HELLP) syndrome.

ALTERATION IN COAGULATION FACTORS (OTHER THAN PLATELETS) AND PROCOAGULANTS

Although thrombocytopenia is one major contributor to hypocoagubility in pre-eclampsia, many other factors add up to this state. Fibrinogen plays a big role in this. Physiologically in normal pregnancies fibrinogen levels rise. These levels can reach 800 mg/dL. But with the development of pre-eclampsia and accidental haemorrhage, fibrinogen levels tend to fall. In pre-eclampsia, the entire maternal vasculature has fibrin deposition all along its endothelial surface. It is a result of an immunological process leading to massive consumption of fibrinogen which ultimately gets converted to fibrin. This low-key but extensive coagulation process that is found in the entire maternal vasculature leads to hypofibrinogenemia.

Normal pregnancy is a hypercoagulable state. In non-pregnant states, fibrinogen can physiologically rise to 400 mg/dL. In pregnancy, these levels can even rise to 800 mg/dL. This can have a bearing on clinical decision making. In clinical practice,

levels less than 150 mg/dL can be accompanied by bleeding and, if less than 100 mg/dL, can indicate a life-threatening emergency. However, in clinical practice, decision making based on absolute levels can be tricky. In a woman who has her pregnancy levels of fibrinogen rise to 800 mg/dL, waiting for levels to drop to 200 mg/dL for intervention could be dangerous. If levels of fibrinogen before the onset of pre-eclampsia are known, it is prudent to label a woman as having hypofibrinogenemia if the levels are reduced to half or more.

ALTERATION IN OTHER CELLULAR COMPONENTS OF BLOOD

Extensive changes (up to 74%) in the shape of the RBCs have been reported in pre-eclampsia.[1] The peripheral smear of a woman with pre-eclampsia can show cells like schizocytes, spherocytes, reticulocytes, etc. Schizocytes are the most commonly seen. They can be found in as high as 39% of women with pre-eclampsia.[1] The commonest and consistent reason for these alterations in the shape of RBCs is attributed to the endothelial damage. It can mechanically deform and haemolyze erythrocytes as they pass through the capillaries. These changes can be rarely associated with haemoglobinuria.

Another feature of ongoing haemolysis is the development of jaundice. It is interesting to note that although RBCs are more fragile in pre-eclampsia, jaundice does not appear so readily. The only explanation for this is the fact that hepatic function tends to remain unaffected to a considerable degree in pre-eclampsia. It appears that the liver can handle the increased load of metabolites resulting from haemolysis. As the disease process advances and the maternal condition rapidly deteriorate, the liver competence also breaks down and jaundice appears. As expected, the rise is in the prehepatic component of bilirubinaemia. One possible reason for the liver being able to handle the increased load of haemolysis could be the anatomical double blood supply that the liver has. Few body organs have double blood supply in the human body. As a result, despite vasospasm and consequent challenge to the organ systems in pre-eclampsia, the liver can handle the load much more efficiently.

REVIEW OF COAGULATION ALTERATIONS IN PRE-ECLAMPSIA

It is well-known that the entire coagulation process gets greatly challenged in pre-eclampsia. Normal uncomplicated human pregnancy is a hypercoagulant state as a result of which blood tends to coagulate more readily in pregnancy. The hypercoagulability of blood during pregnancy has been confirmed with thromboelastography and is thought to be mainly the result of the increased production of factor VII and fibrinogen.[2] It is a protective change. Every pregnant woman is likely to bleed in variable amounts during the process of parturition. This is countered most of the time effectively by the changes in the coagulation system of the woman. The fact that few pregnant women with pre-eclampsia develop coagulation disorders shows that the changes that render the blood hypercoagulable are effective in their purpose.

PLATELETS IN NORMAL AND PRE-ECLAMPTIC PREGNANCIES

The occurrence of thrombocytopenia in 5% of pregnant women at delivery, described as gestational thrombocytopenia, is well documented. A commonly believed concept is that gestational thrombocytopenia is the result of gradually decreasing platelet counts in all women during pregnancy.[3] It is also noteworthy that even if the circulating platelet counts get reduced in pregnancy, the neonatal circulating platelets remain by and large unaffected.

One interesting observation found that circulating platelet levels fell in the early stages of pre-eclampsia. This was concurrently matched with a rise in uric acid levels in the woman's body.[4] This observation was unique because it establishes one important correlation: Uric acid levels in the body reflect oxidative stress. It is known to be one of the strongest reducing systems in the body. Rising levels of uric acid mean ongoing and even accelerated phenomena of oxidative stress in the body. When this is coupled with falling levels of platelets, the correlation can be well understood. Platelets are known to undergo a process of activation. This process of platelet activation is critical and precedes the clinical manifestations of pre-eclampsia. Therefore, rising levels of urate getting coupled with falling levels of platelets indicate that the two, oxidative stress and platelet activation, are coupled in the aetiopathology of pre-eclampsia.

Obstetricians dealing with high-risk patients routinely get a coagulation profile done in women with pre-eclampsia or eclampsia. This may not be always necessary. Tests like the estimation of PT and APTT should be limited to subjects who have platelet counts <100,000/dL. Coagulation indices will change only after platelets have fallen below this.

It has been found that the size of the platelets in circulation during the process of severe pre-eclampsia and eclampsia is larger. The mean platelet volume increases gradually in pregnant women affected by pre-eclampsia compared with women with normal pregnancies. A meta-analysis based on outcomes reported from 50 studies that included 14,614 women showed that the mean platelet volume was significantly higher in women with pre-eclampsia than women without pre-eclampsia.[5] Increase in the size of platelets seems to be occurring irrespective of numerical alterations. Platelets with more mean volume are younger platelets. Therefore, the increase in size reflects the process of platelet mobilisation occurring at a much faster speed in pre-eclampsia.

One more change that has been well documented and hints strongly at the process of platelet activation in pre-eclampsia is the process of platelet degranulation. Before the clinical manifestations of pre-eclampsia manifest, there is a rise in circulating levels of β-thromboglobulin by about 4 weeks.[6] β-thromboglobulin is also called "pro-platelet basic protein". It is a protein that is stored in alpha-granules of platelets and released in large amounts after platelet activation. There is a direct correlation between the rise in β-thromboglobulin levels and degranulation of platelets. Also, platelet degranulation suggests an ongoing process of platelet activation. This process begins early in pre-eclampsia. It may occur even before clinical manifestations of milder forms of the disease appear.

CONCEPT OF COMPETENCE ALTERATION (EFFICIENCY) OF PLATELETS

One interesting feature of thrombocytopenia in pregnancy was demonstrated by Kelton et al.[7] In their published study of women with severe pre-eclampsia, they showed that even if platelet levels are normal, bleeding time can get prolonged. It seems that even if the platelets are numerically unaffected they are decreased in competence in pre-eclampsia.

Most of the markers in modern medical science are expressed on the basis of numerical value. This means that if that particular cell concentration or a particular enzyme or hormone level is high, then the underlying process is active. To make this clear, a linear rise in the number of neutrophils indicates an acute infection. Similarly, a linear rise in levels of transaminases indicates deteriorating liver function. But this concept may be only partially accurate. Although rising neutrophils indicates a higher mobilisation of these leucocytes in the presence of acute infections, it is also true that the neutrophils become more efficient in their working in the presence of acute infection. It is quite likely that an increase in the number and competence both are essential for combating the acute infection. It is possible that a raised count of neutrophil to 13,000 per dL of blood may be shooting up to 20,000–25,000 had their competence too not improved concurrently.

Studies by Kelton et al. could be a pointer to this phenomenon of competence.[7] Rise in bleeding time in absence of significant fall in circulating levels of thrombocytes indicates that in the presence of pre-eclampsia the competence of platelets gets compromised. As a result, their levels on haematological investigations do not reduce, but bleeding time increases. This concept of competency evaluation and competence alteration opens up many exciting possibilities of understanding disease processes and their laboratory parameters in a totally different light.

Although laboratory parameters peg a level of 150,000/dL to be at the lower limit of normal, most pregnant women do not bleed until the platelet levels sink to <50,000/dL in clinical practice. A study by Laskin et al. showed that a platelet count $<100 \times 10^9/L$ is associated with an increased risk of abnormal coagulation and maternal adverse outcomes in women with pre-eclampsia. However, this group expressly states that platelet count should not be used in isolation to guide care because of its poor sensitivity. Whether a platelet count is normal should not be used to determine whether further coagulation tests are needed.[8] This is quite likely an indicator that although the circulating platelet levels are reducing, it may not reflect clinically as bleeding. This is probably because as the levels of platelets start going down, their competence increases. So even a smaller group of platelets are able to hold on and not let bleeding occur.

PLATELET ACTIVATION AND THROMBOXANE A$_2$ PRODUCTION

While explaining the aetiopathogenesis of pre-eclampsia it has been stressed that an unabated oxidative process leads to a series of changes which consequently leads to vasospasm. Normal vascular lumen is maintained by a balance between thromboxane (a potent vasoconstrictor) and prostacyclin (a potent vasodilator) as shown in Figure 11.1. This vasospasm is the main villain inviting different manifestations of pre-eclampsia. Thromboxane is a well-known vasoconstrictor. It causes vasospasm by a direct effect on vascular smooth muscles. What increases thromboxane to tilt the balance in its favour? The answer is platelet activation.

Before increased thromboxane production, there is also a reduction in prostacyclin production. This reduction in production is coupled with a reduction in sensitivity to prostacyclin. Reduction in sensitivity is through messengers like cyclic adenosine monophosphate (cAMP). The production, as well as the sensitivity of vascular endothelium to prostacyclin, is reduced which promotes platelet activation.

Platelets are known to have quite a few structural and biochemical characteristics of smooth muscle cells.[9] There seems to be a definite similarity between smooth muscles and platelets in

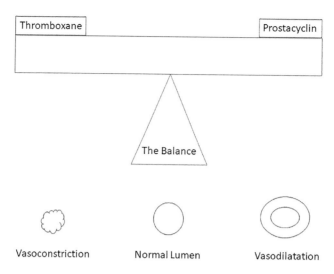

Figure 11.1 The thromboxane-prostacyclin balance.

behaviours and vascular tone. It shows that what is true for platelet behaviour is also true for smooth muscle responses. It explains the similarity in response to the prostacyclin-thromboxane imbalance leading to platelet activation on one hand and an increase in smooth muscle vascular tone on the other. Platelet activation and smooth muscle contraction are not disjointed events. They are two manifestations of the same event. It has also been found that vascular smooth muscle cells stimulate platelets and facilitate thrombus formation.[10] Understanding the similarity between platelets and smooth muscles explains the critical events in the aetiopathogenesis of pre-eclampsia.

REFERENCES

1. Hernández Hernández JD, Villaseñor OR, Del Rio Alvarado J, Lucach RO, Zárate A, Saucedo R, Hernández-Valencia M: Morphological changes of red blood cells in peripheral blood smear of patients with pregnancy-related hypertensive disorders. Arch Med Res 46(6):479–483. doi:10.1016/j.arcmed.2015.07.003.

2. Shreeve NE, Barry JA, Deutsch LR, Gomez K, Kadir RA: Changes in thromboelastography parameters in pregnancy, labor, and the immediate postpartum period. Int J Gynaecol Obstet 134(3):290–293. doi:10.1016/j.ijgo.2016.03.010. Epub 2016 May 26.

3. Reese JA, Peck JD, McIntosh JJ, Vesely SK, George JN: Platelet counts in women with normal pregnancies: A systematic review. Am J Hematol 92(11):1224–1232. doi:10.1002/ajh.24829.

4. Redman C, Bonnar J: Plasma urate changes in pre-eclampsia. Br Med J 1(6125):1484–1485, 1978.

5. Bellos I, Fitrou G, Pergialiotis V, Papantoniou N, Daskalakis G: Mean platelet volume values in preeclampsia: A systematic review and meta-analysis. Pregnancy Hypertens 13:174–180. doi:10.1016/j.preghy.2018.06.016.

6. Belleges V, Spitz B, De Baene L: Platelet activation and vascular damage in gestational hypertension. Am J Obstet Gynecol 166:629–633, 1992.

7. Kelton J, Hunter D, Naema P: A platelet function defect in preeclampsia. Obstet Gynecol 65:107–109, 1995.

8. Laskin S, Payne B, Hutcheon J, Qu Z, Douglas M, Ford J, Lee T, Magee L, von Dadelszen P: The role of platelet counts in

the assessment of inpatient women with preeclampsia. *J Obstet Gynaecol Can* 33(9):900–908, 2011.

9. Baker P, Cunningham F: In Lindheimer M, Roberts J, Cunningham F, editors: *Chesley, Hypertensive Disorders of Pregnancy*, 2nd ed., p. 357, 1998, Stamford, CT, Appleton & Lange.

10. Inoue O, Hokamura K, Shirai T, Osada M, Tsukiji N, Hatakeyama K, et al.: Vascular smooth muscle cells stimulate platelets and facilitate thrombus formation through platelet CLEC-2: Implications in athero-thrombosis. *PLoS One* 10(9):e0139357, 2015. doi:10.1371/journal.pone.0139357. eCollection 2015.

12

Hepatobiliary system

INTRODUCTION

One more vital organ system that bears a heavy brunt of pre-eclampsia is the liver. Epigastric pain, which is one important clinical feature of severe pre-eclampsia, is believed to be hepatic in origin. The stretching of the liver capsule with or without subcapsular haemorrhage is the most likely cause of epigastric pain in pre-eclampsia. HELLP (haemolysis, elevated liver enzymes, low platelet count) syndrome has also been found to have a consistent association with epigastric or right-upper quadrant abdominal pain. Typical clinical symptoms of HELLP syndrome are a pain in the right upper-quadrant abdomen or epigastric pain, nausea and vomiting.[1] Hepatic enzymes are found to be altered consistently in pre-eclampsia in the clinical situation of HELLP syndrome. However, in the absence of this complication of pre-eclampsia, alterations in liver enzymes are not usually found.

Another rare complication of pre-eclampsia is the capsular rupture of the liver. The most common clinical feature of this condition is upper quadrant or epigastric pain. In a review of medical records, only 7 women for a total of 86,858 live births were found to have ruptured subscapular liver hematoma from 2002 to 2015.[2]

PATHOLOGICAL CHANGES IN THE LIVER

It is of interest to know that clinical evidence of liver involvement in pre-eclampsia is not commonly found. Subclinical involvement may be much more. It is known that the liver, heart and the brain are preferred over other systems in the body of a pregnant woman. This is more so when the body faces a crisis as in severe pre-eclampsia or eclampsia. Although it is relatively common to see a compromise in placental and renal functioning in these crisis states, the liver function hardly ever gets clinically compromised. It seems that the liver functioning is given a priority by the double blood supply that this organ has. Consequently, despite a compromise in vascularity of all organs in pre-eclampsia, the liver can withstand this impoverishment much more easily.

Interestingly, early reports of fibroscans of the liver in women with pre-eclampsia show a significant increase in fibrosis of liver tissue. However, there was no difference in liver steatosis between women with pre-eclampsia and women without pre-eclampsia.[3] It appears that this fibrosis must be reversible because no long-term effects have been found on the functioning of the liver in clinical practice.

As stated, subcapsular haemorrhage in women with pre-eclampsia seems to be more consistent with HELLP syndrome. Reports of rupture of subcapsular haematoma appear regularly but not frequently. Some reports of rupture of subcapsular haematoma of the liver are found with Acute Fatty Liver of Pregnancy (AFLP).[4] In one study, 180 cases of hepatic haematoma or rupture were identified: 18 (10.0%) with subcapsular haematoma without hepatic rupture and 162 (90.0%) with capsule rupture.[5]

As regards the gross changes in liver besides subcapsular haemorrhage, petechial haemorrhages have been more consistently found. Their frequency varies from one study to the other. It appears that petechial haemorrhage may be a result of vasospasm-reperfusion damage that occurs in pre-eclampsia. Failure of the hepatic vessels to withstand the pressure of reperfusion seems to cause the vessel walls to break. This may cause petechial haemorrhage, subcapsular haematoma and other haemorrhages in the liver. The extent to which a vessel can withstand the force of the blood depends on its intrinsic capacity. The haemorrhages could be identified if small vessels are involved. If large vessels get disrupted, there could be haematomas. However, on gross examination, besides these changes, the liver remains unaffected.

Description of the pathology of pre-eclampsia would be incomplete if fatty changes in the liver are not touched upon. Vigil-de Gracia and Montufar-Rueda describe the "AFLP triad" in women with acute fatty liver of pregnancy.[6]

In clinical practice, acute fatty liver is diagnosed by an acute deterioration in the condition of the woman with pre-eclampsia. This is combined with a quick rise in liver enzymes and sonographic evidence of acute fatty liver changes. Though these features are consistently found in severe and deteriorating forms of the disease, they are not found in all women consistently. Clinically it appears that AFLP is more fatal than eclampsia.

LIVER IN THE HELLP SYNDROME

The HELLP syndrome is notoriously associated with critical organ systems getting involved along with the liver and can be potentially fatal. It is known to have vicious associations including those with other obstetric vasculopathies like accidental haemorrhage. The kidneys and the cardiovascular systems get readily involved in the HELLP syndrome. It readily complicates into renal failure, pulmonary oedema and subcapsular haemorrhage in the liver. In most instances, delivery is known to improve the condition of the woman. Yet there is a small percentage of women in whom the clinical situation may worsen in the postpartum period.

Rapid delivery through caesarean section is also a preferred intervention. But there can be complications of wound haematoma and intraoperative ooze in these women.

The HELLP syndrome has a risk of recurrence rate of up to 12.8% in some studies.[7] An autoimmune basis has been suggested for the causation of the HELLP syndrome. The immunological basis for the HELLP syndrome is likely because there are associated intrauterine growth restriction (IUGR), accidental haemorrhage, stillbirths and preterm deliveries in subsequent pregnancies. Most of these are known as the major manifestations of pre-eclampsia and have a known strong immunological basis.

REFERENCES

1. Dusse LM, Alpoim PN, Silva JT, Rios DR, Brandão AH, Cabral AC: Revisiting HELLP syndrome. *Clin Chim Acta* 451(Pt B):117–120. doi:10.1016/j.cca.2015.10.024.
2. Henríquez-Villaseca MP, Catalán-Barahona A, Lattus-Olmos J, Vargas-Valdebenito K, Silva-Ruz S: Ruptured subscapular liver hematoma in context of HELLP syndrome. *Rev Med Chil* 146(6):753–761. doi:10.4067/s0034-98872018000600753. [Article in Spanish]
3. Frank Wolf M, Peleg D, Kariv Silberstein N, Assy N, Djibre A, Ben-Shachar I: Correlation between changes in liver stiffness and preeclampsia as shown by transient elastography. *Hypertens Pregnancy* 35(4):536–541.
4. Doumiri M, Elombila M, Oudghiri N, Saoud AT: Ruptured subcapsular hematoma of the liver complicating acute fatty liver of pregnancy. *Pan Afr Med J* 19:38. doi:10.11604/pamj.2014.19.38.4009. eCollection 2014. [Article in French]
5. Vigil-De Gracia P, Ortega-Paz L: Pre-eclampsia/eclampsia and hepatic rupture. *Int J Gynaecol Obstet* 118(3):186–189. doi:10.1016/j.ijgo.2012.03.042.

6. Vigil-de Gracia P, Montufar-Rueda C: Acute fatty liver of pregnancy: Diagnosis, treatment, and outcome based on 35 consecutive cases. *J Matern Fetal Neonatal Med* 24(9):1143–1146. doi:10.3109/14767058.2010.531325.

7. Leeners B, Neumaier-Wagner PM, Kuse S, Mütze S, Rudnik-Schöneborn S, Zerres K, Rath W: Recurrence risks of hypertensive diseases in pregnancy after HELLP syndrome. *J Perinat Med* 39(6):673–678. doi:10.1515/JPM.2011.081.

13

Ophthalmic system

INTRODUCTION

Not far in the recent past, women would present in emergency obstetric units with complaints of the dimness of vision. They had some common features; most common being they had hardly taken any antenatal care. Also, they were invariably women with severe pre-eclampsia or impending eclampsia. Many had accompanying epigastric pain – one more ominous sign in severe pre-eclampsia. Sometimes the dimness of vision progressed to frank blindness. Also, it tends to recur in the subsequent pregnancy. Gratefully, these instances are uncommon now.

Established ophthalmic entities associated with (pre)-eclampsia is cortical blindness, serous retinal detachment, Purtscher-like retinopathy, central retinal vein occlusions and retinal or vitreous haemorrhages. Ensuing visual symptoms include blurry vision, diplopia, amaurosis fugax, photopsia and scotomata, including homonymous hemianopia.[1]

The pathogenesis of the Purtscher-like retinopathy is associated with retinal haemorrhages and ischaemia probably as a result of the complement-mediated leukoembolisation of the retinal arterioles. There is a leucocytic aggregation as a response to the activation of the complement.[2] It is a rare complication and is found in but not exclusive to pre-eclampsia.[3]

THE PERIPHERAL PATHOGENESIS OF OPHTHALMIC CHANGES IN PRE-ECLAMPSIA

There are multiple explanations for the ophthalmic features in pre-eclampsia. One of these is peripheral, meaning that the cause is in the retina.

The exudative retinal detachment is a rare cause (<1%) of visual loss in pre-eclampsia and eclampsia, produced by the involvement of the choroidal vascularisation.[2] As is well known, the human retina is a multi-layered structure. The deepest layer of the retina carries on as the optic nerve. In normal non-diseased situations, an image is focused on the superficial layer of the retina. This transmits an electronic impulse down the succeeding layers to the optic nerve. This nerve carries the impulse to the brain. Here the impulse gets sorted out and overturned by 180 degrees. The result is that the human being "sees".

In severe pre-eclampsia, in susceptible women, there occurs a process of retinal oedema. This is a consequence of vasospasm locally followed by reperfusion damage and incompetence of vessel walls. Retinal oedema leads to diffuse separation of retinal layers. This distances the most superficial layer of the retina from the deepest layer. In retinal oedema of severe pre-eclampsia, the image formed does send the signal to the deeper layer. But because of oedema, this impulse gets diluted and fuzzy. Also, the distance between the layers gets increased. As a result of this, the optic nerve gets a weak signal. This depleted or weakened signal leads to a perception of dimness of vision. The separation of retinal layers could be more severe. In such a situation, though the image does form on the superficial layer; it is deep down the impulse just fails to reach the optic nerve. The result is blackout or blindness.

However, these peripheral causes are by and large completely reversible. Once the woman delivers, the retinal oedema is reversed. The oedema also reverses. All layers of the retina fall back to their original state. They are again in close approximation with each other. So the image formed on the superficial layer once again quickly sends the impulse to the optic nerve and the woman starts "seeing" again.

THE CENTRAL PATHOGENESIS OF OPHTHALMIC CHANGES IN PRE-ECLAMPSIA

There are some subjects in whom the visual disturbance does not get completely reversed. These are subjects who have a central cause of visual disturbance. Optic nerve fibres once emerging from the deep layer of the retina goes to the optic chiasma. From the optic chiasma, these fibres pass to the occipital lobe from where they are directed to the anterior brain. In subjects with the central cause of visual disturbances, the cause of visual disturbance is at the occipital lobe. It usually causes permanent damage to nerve fibres here. Unluckily, this central cause does not reverse because the damage is permanent. The women in such a situation may not get the complete restoration of vision. This is because of the central nervous system having an inherent inability to regenerate and repair once injured or destroyed.

VISUAL ALTERATIONS OF SPECIAL MENTION – RECURRENT AND UNILATERAL

Another feature of these visual disturbances in women with imminent eclampsia is a recurrence. It is not uncommon to find such women reporting with first signs of visual alterations to the emergency obstetric care units seeking help. In these women, retinal vasculature has an inherent propensity to develop oedema and subsequent changes. As a result, they develop such features every time there is pre-eclampsia. Indeed in these women, pre-eclampsia is also recurrent. However, visual disturbances can occur much earlier and in more severe forms with each subsequent pregnancy.

One more interesting aspect of blindness in pre-eclampsia is the fact that in some women this visual handicap develops unilaterally. Usually, it is retinal in origin as described and is reversible. As regards the cortical origin of unilateral visual disturbance that is seen in some women with pre-eclampsia, it has been found that the occipital lobe gets principally involved.[4] A recent case report is related to peripartum vision loss, which was reversible and was also associated with partial haemolysis, elevated liver enzymes and low platelets (HELLP) syndrome.[5]

While on ophthalmic changes in severe pre-eclampsia and eclampsia, it is worthwhile to revisit the funduscopic changes in this condition. Metaphorically, it has been stated that retinal vessels reflect the changes in renal and intracranial vessels. It has also been shown that the severity of retinopathy in pre-eclampsia is directly related to the level of placental insufficiency and intrauterine growth restriction (IUGR). The severity of retinopathy might be independent of systemic blood pressure.[6] However, there are three points where funduscopic examination does help in decision making in clinical practice:

- First, it helps to differentiate between chronic hypertension in women developing superimposed pre-eclampsia over women without hypertension.
- Then, worsening changes a fundoscopy on serial assessment in clinical practice helps decide in favour of early intervention.
- Finally, the presence of papilloedema at any stage of pregnancy in a women with pre-eclampsia is an indication for immediate intervention.

In modern times with the advent of colour Doppler, fundoscopy has lost its value. Colour Doppler is better and more versatile in decision-making in obstetric vasculopathies in general and pre-eclampsia in particular.

REFERENCES

1. Roos N, Wiegman M, Jansonius N, Zeeman G: Visual disturbances in (pre)eclampsia. *Obstet Gynecol Surv* 67(4):242–250, 2012.
2. Mihu D, Mihu C, Tălu S, Costin N, Ciuchină S, Măluţan A: Ocular changes in preeclampsia. *Oftalmologia* 52(2):16–22, 2008.

3. Ang LJPS, Chang BCM: Purtscher-like retinopathy—A rare complication of acute myocardial infarction and a review of the literature. *Saudi J Ophthalmol* 31(4):250–256, 2017. doi:10.1016/j.sjopt.2017.05.009.

4. Swende T, Abwa T: Reversible blindness in fulminating preeclampsia. *Ann Afr Med* 8(3):189–191, 2009.

5. Pradeep AV, Rao S, Ramesh Kumar R: Partial HELLP syndrome with unilateral exudative retinal detachment treated conservatively. *Saudi J Ophthalmol* 28(4):329–331, 2014. doi:10.1016/j.sjopt.2014.03.011.

6. Gupta A, Kaliaperumal S, Setia S, Suchi S, Rao V: Retinopathy in preeclampsia: Association with birth weight and uric acid level. *Retina* 28(8):1104–1110, 2008.

14

Renal system

INTRODUCTION

The renal system bears a maximum brunt of the onslaught of the disease process of pre-eclampsia. While the central nervous system (CNS) is protected the most, kidneys seem to be least prioritised of the body protective systems. There can also be some long-term effects and some unfortunate women can end up with renal failure and need dialysis and renal transplant subsequently.

BRIEF OUTLINE OF RENAL CHANGES IN PREGNANCY

As the renal system is the principal player in the process of pre-eclampsia, it will be useful to review the physiological changes in pregnancy. The GFR increases by about 50%. There is a consequent decrease in serum creatinine, plasma urea and blood uric acid levels in normal pregnancy. The kidneys increase in length but not so much in width. There is an increase in kidney volume. Physiological hydronephrosis during pregnancy occurs in 43%–100% pregnant women, and it is more prevalent with the advancing trimester.[1] A rise in serum aldosterone results in a net gain of approximately 1 g of sodium. There is a concomitant rise in progesterone, which protects the pregnant woman from hypokalaemia. The threshold for thirst and antidiuretic hormone secretion are depressed, resulting in lower osmolality and serum sodium levels.[2] The rise in GFR in pregnancy leads to a series of changes, including the most obvious increase in urine output. Increase in blood volume and an increase in renal circulation both contribute to increased urine output. There is more blood to be filtered in pregnancy, and therefore, the renal system goes into an unstressed overdrive.

VULNERABILITY OF RENAL SYSTEM

In pre-eclampsia, the entire competence of the renal system gets challenged. The physiological increase in blood volume in normal pregnancy is either annulled or constricted in pre-eclampsia. Also, in pre-eclampsia, the renal vascular system undergoes vasoconstriction along with the woman's entire vascular system. The kidneys encounter lowered blood volume and vasoconstriction. As a result, they get dangerously vulnerable to getting dried up. The intensity and frequency with which this occurs depend on the severity of pre-eclampsia and the rapidity with which it progresses. It also depends on the inherent robustness of the renal system of each pregnant woman to bear the changes. This gets reflected in varied clinical manifestation of renal system involvement in pre-eclampsia and other obstetric vasculopathies.

Once the precarious balance of blood supply to the renal system is understood, one can understand the grave complications of pre-eclampsia with more ease. In conditions like abruptio placenta with pre-eclampsia, the renal system gets further impoverished of its blood supply. This is like pushing someone who is about to fall. With the added insult of accidental haemorrhage, the kidneys may not be able to bear it any further, and at times, renal failure occurs. In most subjects, the inherent reserve of the renal system can withstand the changes of pre-eclampsia. As a result of this, total renal shut down is not seen often in clinical practice. However, oliguria is consistently seen in pre-eclampsia, especially in pre-eclampsia of a severe type.

One more challenge that the obstetrician faces while managing women with pre-eclampsia is handling the fluid and electrolyte balance.

This challenge is more profound in subjects with severe pre-eclampsia and its complication of accidental haemorrhage. It has been found that when infusions are given to women with pre-eclampsia, the heart goes quickly into an overdrive. It increases the cardiac output by increasing the Left Ventricular Stroke Work Index. This means the left ventricle forces out additional blood. Unluckily in such subjects, the heart is already facing strong resistance from blood vessels that are in vasospasm. Attempts to increase the renal perfusion by increasing the fluid and electrolytes by infusing externally can cause the heart pump to fail. It results in pulmonary oedema and if not corrected properly, even death.

One habit that some practitioners have is trying to combat the renal hypo-efficiency in pre-eclampsia with diuretics. This can also be dangerous because the diuretics will forcibly increase the blood supply to the kidneys. A system which is already impoverished of blood supply is forced to divert blood to the renal system which can prove the proverbial last straw on the camel's back. As a result, the heart could pump still faster and fail much more readily. It is, therefore, desirable to put a central venous pressure line to get an idea of how much fluid to give and when not to give any fluid.

SPECIAL FEATURES OF RENAL FAILURE COMPLICATING PRE-ECLAMPSIA

Accidental haemorrhage is the commonest complication of pre-eclampsia (particularly severe pre-eclampsia). Renal failure is a dreaded occurrence in accidental haemorrhage. The renal failure in accidental haemorrhage complicating pre-eclampsia is more a result of tubular necrosis and less of cortical necrosis. Usually, this is in a ratio of 80:20 for tubular to cortical insult. If prompt and adequate blood transfusions are given to these subjects, renal failure can be reversed or altogether prevented. Resultant long-term effects on the renal system are few.

It is relevant to note that accidental haemorrhage has a notorious habit to recur and also has the complication of renal shut down. Nevertheless, with better monitoring facilities available and better neonatal intensive care, obstetricians tend

to intervene much earlier. This has reduced both complications of pre-eclampsia – accidental haemorrhage as well as its consequential renal failure, significantly. If the obstetric team is not vigilant or if the woman is unable to get quality antenatal care, recurrent renal failure with a poor outcome can still occur.

In 20% of the subjects in whom the cortical necrosis becomes predominant, renal failure is irreversible, warranting a renal transplant and dialysis. In women with persistent albuminuria in severe pre-eclampsia, there is an increased tendency for renal failure. However, the presence of albuminuria may not be indicative of an impending renal shut down. In actuality, it reflects the compromised renal function, the consequence of which is a renal shut down. Thus, proteinuria is not the cause of renal compromise and renal failure, but in actuality, it is a marker of the underlying pathology.

A word about uric acid estimation for assessing renal function in pre-eclampsia will not be out of place here. Although many biochemical markers have been used to assess renal function in non-pregnant women, many of them as seen become incompetent in pregnancy more so in pre-eclampsia. Uric acid assessment in pre-eclampsia has been done at different times to assess renal function. One study concludes that monitoring of plasma creatinine level among patients with pre-eclampsia will help to predict those at risk of developing pre-eclampsia. In the same way, monitoring of plasma uric acid level in those with pre-eclampsia will help to predict those that will develop eclampsia.[3] This indicates worsening of the condition. Here the role of uric acid gets reinforced as a good prognosticator rather than predictor as has been suggested in this study. Uric acid is a strong reducing substance in the body. It has, therefore, a limited role in reflecting the renal function in a woman with pre-eclampsia. When the level of uric acid is assessed, the state of oxidative stress in the pregnant women is being studied and not the renal function. No wonder, a subsequent study found uric acid to be unreliable for assessing renal function in pregnancy.[4] This matter has been dealt with in much greater detail elsewhere (Chapter 4).

The HELLP syndrome is one more condition that can cause renal failure while complicating pre-eclampsia. HELLP is the acronym for haemolysis, elevated hepatic enzymes and low platelets. Some workers have shown that the HELLP syndrome can also occur in absence of pre-eclampsia though its most consistent association is with hypertensive disorders of pregnancy. When the HELLP syndrome is associated with pre-eclampsia, renal failure if it occurs, will be stormy and can be irreversible. This is because, in such combinations, acute cortical necrosis gets precipitated. This is an irreversible and dreaded form of renal failure. A combination of comorbidities like accidental haemorrhage and pre-eclampsia and the HELLP syndrome and pre-eclampsia together accounts for up to 80% of the subjects with pregnancy-related irreversible renal failure.[5,6]

RENAL LESIONS

Pathological changes in the renal system can occur in pre-eclampsia and its complication of accidental haemorrhage, in a big way. In the former, the changes are the result of vasospasm and in the latter because of acute blood loss. Sheehan et al. have done pioneering work in this field, which must be acknowledged and referred to. This team diligently studied and documented renal changes in subjects who died in pregnancy on postmortem. They compared postmortem findings of 112 women without pre-eclampsia who died of hypertensive disorders of pregnancy with those who died of other obstetric causes. They performed postmortems within 2 hours of death, thereby increasing the accuracy of their results. Even after so many years, their results have been corroborated by images obtained through modern imaging technologies. No discussion and pathology of pre-eclampsia or eclampsia is complete without taking into account the description of these workers. The entire compilation of their work has been published in a book by Sheehan and Lynch.[7]

ARE KIDNEY CHANGES IN PRE-ECLAMPSIA – PATHOGNOMONIC?

While one must accept that the kidneys do bear the heavy brunt of the disease of pre-eclampsia, they are not the game changers in the entire aetiopathology of pre-eclampsia. This is important to understand from various angles. Access to the renal system is relatively easy. Also, changes in the renal systems can be easily studied primarily through an easily obtainable urine sample. Changes in renal systems can be relatively easily

viewed because kidney biopsies are not difficult to perform. All this gives an advantage to workers in this field being able to study the kidneys extensively and easily. This is not to run down the involvement of kidneys in pre-eclampsia and its complications. They do bear a heavy brunt. But the ease of access to kidneys lends great importance to renal changes in pre-eclampsia. So much so that renal changes were described as pathognomonic of pre-eclampsia. Also, there were suggestions that the aetiopathology of pre-eclampsia and its complications lies in the kidneys. In short, renal changes seem to have got overhyped.

It is well-known now that not the kidneys but the foetomaternal interface is at the core of the aetiopathology in pre-eclampsia. Changes emanating here involve other organs including the kidneys and systems in their processes secondarily. Until recently, science did not have an accurate and reliable means to know what is happening at the foetomaternal interface. As a result, the kidneys, which were easily accessible, got studied extensively. With the advent of ultrasonography in general and colour Doppler in particular the picture changed. Imaging of what is happening at the foetomaternal interface is now possible. As a result, the accurate picture of aetiopathology became clear to the scientific investigators. We now have a reasonably precise idea of what all causes and what is the sequence of events in pre-eclampsia.

GROSS CHANGES IN THE KIDNEYS

While examining the pathology it can be traditionally divided into gross and microscopic appearance. Microscopic appearance can be further divided into light microscopic appearance and appearance under electron microscopic. As regards the gross appearance of kidneys in pre-eclampsia, there is an insignificant increase in the size of the kidneys. On cut section, the kidneys appear pale and have a relatively enlarged cortex. However, compared to gross changes, microscopic changes are for more extensive.

ON MICROSCOPY

The glomeruli are enlarged and solidified ("bloodless") as a result of narrowed or occluded capillary lumens that are the result of swelling of the native endothelial cells and, to a lesser extent, mesangial cells. Glomerular volume is increased and correlates with the severity of the disease.[8] Thrombosis by light microscopy is decidedly unusual, although fibrin can be detected by immunofluorescence in glomeruli. In marked contrast, in non-pre-eclamptic Thrombotic Microangiopathies (TMA), thrombosis of vessels or glomeruli is a central finding.[8] TMA is a pathology that results in thrombosis in capillaries and arterioles because of an endothelial injury.[9] It may be seen in association with thrombocytopaenia, anaemia, purpura, and renal failure.

Lesions of pre-eclampsia share some similarities with and intriguing differences from those of non-preeclamptic TMA, likely owing to their differing pathogenesis.[10] The immunofluorescence findings are somewhat variable with fibrin deposition often being a prominent feature. The low-level glomerular Ig deposition in severe pre-eclampsia, reported by some, probably represents non-immunologic insudation. This conclusion is supported by the ultrastructural observation that electron-dense deposits are inconspicuous. Its chief diagnostic role lies in excluding immune complex glomerulonephritis, such as lupus nephritis, which often flares during pregnancy.[4]

Old references have described some of these changes as glomerular nephropathy. Typically characterised by glomerular hypertrophy and decreased glomerular space as a result of swelling of glomerular endothelium, there is an increased capillary wall thickness without significant changes in glomerular cellularity. From the description of Sheehan et al., it seems that an increase in glomerular size could be a result of a response to falling renal circulation due to vasospasm in pre-eclampsia.[7] While the blood supply reduces, kidneys make internal arrangements to make their work more competent.

Cellular alterations in the kidneys reflect the attempts made by the kidneys to improve its functioning in the face of impoverished blood supply in developing pre-eclampsia. There is an increased proliferation of the mesangial and endothelial cells. Though these cells have been shown to proliferate, the increase in cellularity is numerically minimal.

One of the characteristic features of pre-eclampsia is what is described as "bloodless glomeruli". These are obstructed hypovascular appearance of the glomeruli tufts. Narrowing of the glomerular capillary loops reflecting the generalised process of vasospasm is also consistently found. Endothelial hypertrophy, a characteristic feature of the microvascular pathology of pre-eclampsia, is partly responsible for the compromise of the vascular spaces in the glomeruli.[11]

One more feature ascribed to pre-eclampsia in the kidneys is the presence of foam cells. This so-called foamy appearance of some cells is a reflection of characteristic alterations in the cytoplasm showing the presence of clear vacuoles and lipid droplets. When the cytoplasm is displaced by massive intracellular lipid deposits, the cells acquire a foamy appearance and so are called "foam cells".[12] Currently, the presence of foam cells is believed to indicate the process of acute atherosis in pre-eclampsia. It can be found even in spiral arterioles in the decidua. Acute atherosis also occurs in other pregnancy complications, even in normal pregnancies.[13]

There was once a belief that mobilisation of fat to enter the cytoplasm and generation of foam cells is a marker of a crisis. It was believed to show that the organ system is challenged and its own existence is at risk. This was when electron microscopy had still not made its appearance. With electron microscopic studies becoming available, more sensitive and minute pictures became known to science. It is now possible to detect even tiny amounts of fat mobilisation and deposition on the glomeruli. It became evident that the presence of intra-glomerular foam cells does not necessarily represent a terminal event. It just shows the evolution of the disease.

The reported frequency of intraglomerular foam cells is quite variable. It can vary between 4% and 35%, depending on the timing of the biopsy, method of tissue processing and staining and the sensitivity of the technique used to detect the presence of intra-glomerular fat cells.[12,14]

One more change reported from studies of renal biopsies that have created lots of confusion and debate is the presence of capillary wall thickening in the tuft of glomerular capillaries. This was erroneously labelled as "membranous glomerulonephritis". With the technological advances, it was found that the presence of capillary wall thickening in the glomeruli is merely a reflection of the severity of the disease and nothing beyond. Other capillary loop pathologies have also been described in the literature.

These include the so-called "cigar-shaped loops", "ballooned loops", "Pouting", etc. These appear in some references at different periods of time. However, their clinical bearing, as well as bearing on the understanding of aetiopathology, is at the most limited.

Sheehan has described classical changes in glomerular mesangium in pre-eclampsia. He has described it as a peculiar change in the mesangium, commonly associated with the healing stage of the disease. It is characterised by vacuolation of the mesangial stalks resembling a "string of beads".[14] In the same reference, Sheehan has further mentioned that various mesangial lesions described are usually focal in nature. Approximately, 8% of the subjects associated with a severe form of the disease manifest a generalised dilatation of the mesangium and distortion of capillary loops.

Two more lesions that have been described in the kidneys of patients affected by pre-eclampsia are focal segmental glomerular sclerosis (FSGS) and its variants described as early cellular lesions or glomerular tip lesions. The clinical bearing of these lesions is unknown, and therefore, they remain by and large confined to the realms of pathology books of the disease. Podocyte loss is the fundamental basis of glomerulosclerosis. FSGS is a progressive glomerular disease, and its glomerular features are a prototype of podocyte loss-driven glomerulosclerosis. The glomerular pathology of FSGS is characterised by a focal and segmental location of the sclerotic lesions in human FSGS; segmental sclerosis often shows simultaneous intra- and extra-capillary changes, including parietal cell migration, capillary collapse, hyaline deposition, intra-capillary thrombi and occasional hypercellularity. This suggests that local cellular events, initiated by podocyte loss, are the basis of the segmental lesions in FSGS.[15]

The scientists who tried to study the clinicopathological correlation between FSGS and pre-eclampsia tried to study the clinical course of the disease, resolution and long-term consequences in subjects with FSGS. No such correlation was found. It seems that subjects with FSGS are not having a more severe form of the disease; they do not have a poorer or better obstetric outcome; and they tend to reverse the changes of pre-eclampsia as early or as late as those subjects who do not show FSGS.

Gabel et al. beautifully summarised this entire controversy regarding the clinical importance, if any, with FSGS. They state that localised lesions resembling those of FSGS are identified in approximately 20% subjects who have a clinical diagnosis of pre-eclampsia. To date, as stated by them, there is no evidence that this subset of patients will have long-term renal dysfunction, albeit they may present with atypical or severe pre-eclampsia.[16]

RENAL FUNCTION ALTERATIONS IN PRE-ECLAMPSIA

As has been made amply clear, alterations in renal function are profound in pre-eclampsia. Also, the renal system is not on a priority list of the pregnant woman when she faces a crisis. Therefore, pathological alterations get all the more amplified. Compensatory processes in renal systems for a crisis are present, but once they crash, the renal systems get handsomely beaten up. Besides these, the renal system is relatively easily accessible to the investigating scientific community. Urine is easy to procure and profusely available. Also, renal biopsy is easily doable with some experience. Thus, functional and structural alterations can be studied with relative ease. By 1998, 23 groups had already published their studies on renal changes in pre-eclampsia as has been tabulated by Conrad and Lindheimer in 1998.[17]

Hormonal changes during pregnancy allow for increased blood flow to the kidneys and altered autoregulation such that GFR increases significantly through reductions in net glomerular oncotic pressure and increased renal size. The mechanisms for maintenance of increased GFR change through the trimesters of pregnancy, continuing into the postpartum period. Important causes of pregnancy-specific renal dysfunction have been further studied, but much needs to be learned.[18] The most consistent physiological alteration reported in most of the studies is the significant reduction in the GFR and effective renal plasma flow (ERPF) in pre-eclampsia.[19] In all of these studies, about a 30%–35% reduction in these two parameters emerges consistently.

Vasospasm, which has been stressed, restressed and probably overstressed in these pages understandably leads to a reduction in blood flow of the renal system. Also, the blood volume in a woman with pre-eclampsia is constricted in comparison to the woman without pre-eclampsia at same pregnancy duration. Both of these produce a reduction in effective blood flow through the kidneys, which in turn leads to a reduction in GFR and ERPF. Indeed other mechanisms also contribute to the alterations like the vascular endothelial damage that occurs in pre-eclampsia. However, this and allied glomerular dysfunctions reported are also a result of organ hypoperfusion found in pre-eclampsia and therefore, subsequent effects.

Post-delivery, GFR improves most consistently within the first week to 10 days. Renal functions recover much faster than the structural recovery. GFR recovery is most notable. ERPF recovery occurs slowly. This is reflected through the recovery in GFR outstripping the recovery in ERPF, which, in turn, is outstripping the recovery on renal biopsy changes.

RENAL HANDLING OF PROTEINS IN PRE-ECLAMPSIA

Two clinical features of pre-eclampsia make one inquisitive to know how the kidneys handle proteins in pre-eclampsia. These two features are albuminuria and oedema. The intravascular mass of albumin showed no change between the non-pregnant state and up to about 12 weeks of pregnancy. But there was a significant rise of 19.5% between 12 and 28 weeks of gestation, an overall increase of 19%. However, the extravascular albumin mass tends to decline.[20] As a result, the fluid tends to get held back in the intravascular channels. Any alteration in this relationship between intravascular albumin mass and its extravascular distribution tends to release the fluids held on by the albumin. The clinical result of this is oedema. It is possible that oestradiol or progesterone together may mediate in the reduced synthesis of albumin.

Urinary protein excretion is increased during normal pregnancy as has been widely known. This is studied in great detail using different positions occupied by the gravida as well as the timing of the day, such as urinary protein excretion in the night compared with excretion during the day. It is also of interest to note that the alteration in this urinary function of protein excretion is not restored to pre-pregnant stage until 16 weeks to 1 year postpartum.

Similarly, other proteins like low-molecular proteins and enzymes are also excreted in increased amount during normal pregnancy. The proximate tubular resorption is reduced in normal pregnancy. This restores faster after pregnancy compared to the excretory changes in the kidneys.

Handling of urinary excretion of proteins in pre-eclampsia

Serum albumin, as well as low-molecular-weight proteins like immunoglobulin G (IgG), is decreased in circulation in pre-eclampsia as has been shown in many studies.[21] It seems that the overall disposition of the kidneys is such that in pre-eclampsia there is an increased loss of proteins, especially albumin. This is coupled by incompetent resorption of excreted proteins through the glomerular membrane. It seems that the electronic disposition of the glomerular membrane also plays an important role in these changes, which ultimately predisposes a woman with pre-eclampsia to develop albuminuria. When and at what stage of pregnancy this excretion does become apparent on laboratory reports is difficult to predict. But by a rule of thumb, it appears that the increasing severity of pre-eclampsia makes albumin and other proteins more easily apparent in the urine of women with pre-eclampsia.

RENIN-ANGIOTENSIN SYSTEM IN PRE-ECLAMPSIA

It has been postulated that angiotensin-II may play an essential role in the pathogenesis of pre-eclampsia. In a transgenic mouse model, the mice developed pregnancy-associated hypertension (PAH) by the overproduction of angiotensin-II in maternal circulation during late pregnancy. The mice with PAH exhibited maternal and foetal abnormalities, such as proteinuria, cardiac hypertrophy, placental morphological changes and IUGR. In one study, to attenuate the activity of redundant renin-angiotensin system during the advanced stages of PAH, olmesartan an angiotensin receptor blocker, was administered, as was captopril, an angiotensin-converting enzyme inhibitor, from 17 to 19 days of gestation, and evaluated for their effects on cardiac and placental abnormalities and foetal growth. Olmesartan and captopril administration lowered the blood pressure of mice with PAH, and placental histological change and severe IUGR were markedly ameliorated in both groups. On the contrary, both treatments had little effect on cardiac remodelling during the advanced stages of PAH. These findings highlight a variety of therapeutic actions of the renin angiotensin system repression on the progressive pathology of PAH in mice.[22]

REFERENCES

1. Faúndes A, Brícola-Filho M, Pinto e Silva JL: Dilatation of the urinary tract during pregnancy: Proposal of a curve of maximal caliceal diameter by gestational age. *Am J Obstet Gynecol* 178(5):1082–1086, 1998.
2. Cheung KL, Lafayette RA: Renal physiology of pregnancy. *Adv Chronic Kidney Dis* 20(3):209–214, 2013. doi:10.1053/j.ackd.2013.01.012.
3. Wakwe V, Abudu O: Estimation of plasma uric acid in pregnancy induced hypertension (PIH). Is the test still relevant? *Afr J Med Sci* 28(3–4):155–158, 1999.
4. Salako B, Odukogbe A, Olayemi O, Adedapo K, Aimakhu C, Alu F, Ola B: Serum albumin, creatinine, uric acid and hypertensive disorders of pregnancy. *East Afr Med J* 80(8):424–428, 2003.
5. Gurrieri C, Garovic VD, Gullo A, Bojanić K, Sprung J, Narr B, Weingarten T: Kidney injury during pregnancy: Associated comorbid conditions and outcomes. *Arch Gynecol Obstet* 286(3):567–573, 2012.
6. Ahonen J, Nuutila M: HELLP syndrome—Severe complication during pregnancy. *Duodecim* 128(6):569–577, 2012.
7. Sheehan H, Lynch J: *Pathology of Toxemia of Pregnancy*: Baltimore, 1973, p. 807, Williams & Wilkins.
8. Tsokos M, Longauer F, Kardosová V, Gavel A, Anders S, Schulz F: Maternal death in pregnancy from HELLP syndrome. A report of three medico-legal autopsy cases with special reference to distinctive histopathological alterations. *Int J Legal Med* 116(1):50–53, 2002.
9. Benz K, Amann K: Thrombotic microangiopathy: New insights. *Curr Opin Nephrol Hypertens* 19(3):242–247. doi:10.1097/MNH.0b013e3283378f25.
10. Stillman I, Karumanchi S: The glomerular injury of preeclampsia. *J Am Soc Nephrol* 18(8):2281–2284, 2007.
11. Eremina V, Sood M, Haigh J, Nagy A, Lajoie G, Ferrara N, Gerber H, Kikkawa Y, Miner J, Quaggin S: Glomerular-specific alterations of VEGF-A expression lead to distinct congenital and acquired renal diseases. *J Clin Invest* 111(5):707–716, 2003.
12. Ogino S: An electron microscopic study of the glomerular alterations of pure-preeclampsia. *Nihon Jinzo Gakkai Shi* 41(4):413–429, 1999.
13. Staff AC, Redman CW: IFPA Award in placentology lecture: Preeclampsia, the decidual battleground and future maternal cardiovascular disease. *Placenta* 35(Suppl):S26–S31. doi:10.1016/j.placenta.2013.12.003. Epub 2013 Dec 18.
14. Sheehan H: Renal morphology in preeclampsia. *Kidney Int* 18:241–252, 1980.
15. Nagata M, Kobayashi N, Hara S: Focal segmental glomerulosclerosis: Why does it occur segmentally? *Pflugers Arch* 469(7–8):983–988, 2017. doi:10.1007/s00424-017-2023-x. Epub 2017 Jun 29.
16. Gabel L, Spargo B, Lindheimer M: The nephrology of preeclampsia. In Tisher C, Brenner B, editors: *Renal Pathology*, 2nd ed., pp. 419–441, 1994, Philadelphia, PA, Lippincott.
17. Conrad K, Lindheimer M: Renal and cardiovascular abnormalities. In Lindheimer M, Roberts J, Cunningham F, editors: *Chesley, Hypertensive Disorders of Pregnancy*, 2nd, p. 280, Table 8.1, 1998, Stamford, CT, Appleton & Lange.
18. Hussein W, Lafayette RA: Renal function in normal and disordered pregnancy. *Curr Opin Nephrol Hypertens* 23(1):46–53, 2014. doi:10.1097/01.mnh.0000436545.94132.52.Ш; Liu X, Zhou Z, Cao Y, Wang B, Xu G: Contributions of blood pressure to proteinuria and renal function in the puerperium. *Blood Press* 18(6):362–366, 2009.
19. Lafayette R, Druzin M, Sibley R, Derby G, Malik T, Huie P, Polhemus C, Deen W, Myers B: Nature of glomerular dysfunction in preeclampsia. *Kidney Int* 54(4):1240–1209, 1998.

20. Whittaker PG, Lind T: The intravascular mass of albumin during human pregnancy: A serial study in normal and diabetic women. *Br J Obstet Gynaecol* 100(6):587–592, 1993.

21. Benoit J, Rey É: Preeclampsia: Should plasma albumin level be a criterion for severity? *J Obstet Gynaecol Can* 33(9):922–926, 2011.

22. Ishimaru T, Ishida J, Nakamura S, Hashimoto M, Matsukura T, Nakamura A, Kunita S, Sugiyama F, Yagami K, Fukamizu A: Short-term suppression of the renin-angiotensin system in mice associated with hypertension during pregnancy. *Mol Med Report* 6(1):28–32, 2012.

PART 6

Clinical features of pre-eclampsia

15

Clinical features

INTRODUCTION

Pre-eclampsia is a disease characterised by hypertension as a cardinal feature. It may be accompanied by proteinuria and or oedema. There are a series of other clinical features that may accompany hypertension as per the severity of the condition as well as the type of pre-eclampsia.

CLASSIFICATION

The ISSHP classification is currently found to be the most popular and most consistently quoted[1]:

1. *Hypertension* in pregnancy may be chronic (pre-dating pregnancy or diagnosed before 20 weeks of pregnancy) or de novo (either pre-eclampsia or gestational hypertension).
2. *Chronic hypertension* is associated with adverse maternal and foetal outcomes and is best managed by tightly controlling maternal blood pressure (110–140/85 mmHg), monitoring foetal growth and repeatedly assessing for the development of pre-eclampsia and maternal complications. This can be done in an outpatient setting.
3. *White-coat hypertension* refers to elevated office or clinic blood pressure ($\geq$140/90 mmHg) but normal blood pressure measured at home or work (<135/85 mmHg); it is not an entirely benign condition and conveys an increased risk for pre-eclampsia.
4. *Masked hypertension* is another form of hypertension, more difficult to diagnose, characterised by blood pressure that is normal at a clinic or office visit but elevated at other times,

most typically diagnosed by 24 hours ambulatory blood pressure monitoring (ABPM) or automated home blood pressure monitoring (HBPM).

5. *Gestational hypertension* is hypertension arising de novo after 20 weeks' gestation in the absence of proteinuria and without biochemical or haematological abnormalities. It is usually not accompanied by foetal growth restriction. Outcomes in pregnancies complicated by gestational hypertension are normally good, but about a quarter of women with gestational hypertension (particularly those who present at <34 weeks) will progress to pre-eclampsia and have poorer outcomes.
6. *Pre-eclampsia* is a complex medical disorder; worldwide, each year, it is responsible for more than 500,000 foetal and neonatal deaths and over 70,000 maternal deaths. Pre-eclampsia can deteriorate rapidly and without warning; we do not recommend classifying it as "mild" or "severe". The haemolysis, elevated liver enzymes, low platelets, or HELLP syndrome is one (serious) manifestation of pre-eclampsia and not a separate disorder.
7. *Proteinuria* is not mandatory for a diagnosis of pre-eclampsia. Rather, this is diagnosed by the presence of de novo hypertension after 20 weeks' gestation accompanied by proteinuria or evidence of maternal acute kidney injury, liver dysfunction, neurological features, haemolysis or thrombocytopenia or foetal growth restriction. Pre-eclampsia may develop or be recognised for the first time intrapartum or early postpartum in some cases.

HYPERTENSION

It is now agreed that any pregnant subject who registers a blood pressure of 130 systolic and/or 90 diastolic in pregnancy taken on two consecutive readings 6 hours apart after adequate rest of at least half an hour is hypertensive. Although this definition uses both systolic as well as diastolic blood pressure, MAP is considered to make things easy. The MAP is calculated with both these indices together. As is well-known, MAP is the diastolic pressure plus one-third the pulse pressure. A MAP of 103 and above taken after adequate bed rest (or at least half an hour) on two consecutive readings at least 6 hours apart is considered indicative of hypertension. As such, many authorities recommend using the MAP in severe pre-eclampsia protocols, with 125 mmHg being the most commonly used cut-off point.[2] When blood pressure is measured in the first or second trimester of pregnancy, the MAP is a better predictor for pre-eclampsia than systolic blood pressure, diastolic blood pressure or an increase of blood pressure.[3]

In labelling a women as hypertensive in pregnancy, many controversies have expectedly arisen. One such controversy is the cut-off of 130/90 mmHg. At times, it does happen that a woman may show changes in hypertension in pregnancy before those levels are reached. This usually happens in diminutive subjects whose basal blood pressure itself is very low. Many pregnant Indian women have their normal systolic blood pressure hovering around 100 and diastolic blood pressure hovering around 64–70. In them, to wait for the blood pressure to reach the threshold of 130/90 may be late and even dangerous. Also, a subject usually shows a fall in blood pressure during mid-trimester. This can further reduce an already low blood pressure of in pregnancy. It is not unusual to find subjects with a normal basal blood pressure of 90/65 (average) at mid-trimester in India.

Does this require redefining hypertension? The answer to this is no. It is not necessary to redefine hypertension. It is better to add a further specification, which makes situations easy and broadly encompassing to handle. It is, therefore, added that if any pregnant woman who registers a rise of 30 mmHg in her systolic and/or 15 mmHg in her diastolic blood pressure to her known basal blood pressure should be labelled hypertensive. The rider that this blood pressure is to be recorded after adequate bed rest of at least half an hour holds for all. Also, the rider that these blood pressure readings should be taken at least 6 hours apart also holds. Thus, if a subject has a basal blood pressure set at 94/68 mmHg in a given situation, for her blood pressure of 124/83 mmHg and above can be labelled as hypertensive.

This addition can act as a double-edged sword. It can prove to be an advantage for the fact that many subjects who may be missed as hypertensive can be brought under care. On the flip side, is that if the basal blood pressure of the subject is not known, this definition may become inapplicable. Nevertheless, there will still be 5% or fewer subjects at maximum who may be under- or over-diagnosed as hypertensive with these two definition facets. Therefore, for a clinician, most of the times 130/90 mmHg (MAP: 103) or a rise of 30 mmHg systolic or 15 mmHg diastolic should suffice to label a pregnant woman hypertensive.

PROTEINURIA

Proteinuria is not essential for the diagnosis of pre-eclampsia but is related to the severity of the disease and adverse foetal outcomes.[4] Conventionally, proteinuria is calibrated as a presence of 100 mg/dL of albumin in spot urine samples taken at least 6 hours apart. Alternatively, it is quantified as the presence of 300 mg/dL of albumin in 24-hours urine sample of the pregnant woman. Currently, however, the dipstick method has replaced these two in clinical practice. For the test, a strip of chemically treated paper is placed into the urine. The dipstick changes colour if albumin is present in the urine. Proteinuria is always indicative of albuminuria in communications related to pre-eclampsia until otherwise specified. It usually develops late in the course of the disease. Fascinatingly, absence of proteinuria in presence of severe pre-eclampsia was considered as indicating bad prognosis. Presence of protein (albumin) in urine has been known to be one of the most consistent features of pre-eclampsia. By and large, it reflects upon the extent of renal involvement in the process.

With the advent of colour Doppler in the armamentarium of pre-eclampsia management, investigative parameters like proteinuria lost their importance in day-to-day practice for critical decision making. As stated, the presence of protein in urine is indicative of the extent of renal involvement in the disease process, and renal involvement indicates the extent of systemic involvement in the disease process. This explains the importance of proteinuria.

OEDEMA

Once popular but one of the most unreliable clinical features of pre-eclampsia is oedema. The manifestations of oedema in pre-eclampsia are diverse.[5] This feature has indeed lost its popularity because of this unreliability and is now no more considered amongst the major features of pre-eclampsia. Also, oedema does not indicate the severity of the underlying pathology in any way. A woman may have a mild form of the disease and still have a severe degree of oedema. At the same time, a woman may have severe pre-eclampsia or may even have an eclamptic convulsion and she may have mild oedema. In the absence of reliability, therefore, many times oedema is mentioned as a feature of pre-eclampsia only to complete the list.

Weight gain is another unreliable feature linked with oedema. A pregnant woman is expected to gain about 10 kg of weight by the time she reaches term. To make it simple, she gains weight at the rate of 0, −1, +1, +4, +4, +5, +5, +3, +3 lb/month of her 9 months of pregnancy sequentially. Excessive weight gain was considered as an indicator of developing pre-eclampsia.

GRADES OF SEVERITY OF PRE-ECLAMPSIA

Just like many other conditions in obstetrics, scientists have tried to grade pre-eclampsia as mild, moderate and severe. However, over a period of time only two grades of pre-eclampsia seem to exist: Mild and severe.

Mild pre-eclampsia is diagnosed when:
- Pregnancy is <20 weeks
- Blood pressure is <140 systolic or 90 diastolic
- 0.3 g of protein is collected in a 24-hours urine sample or persistent 1+ protein measurement on urine dipstick
- There are no other signs of problems with the mother or the baby

Severe pre-eclampsia is labelled when:
- Very high blood pressure (<160 systolic or 110 diastolic)
- More than 5 g of protein in a 24-hours sample
- Signs of central nervous system problems (a severe headache, blurry vision, altered mental status)
- Signs of liver problems (nausea and/or vomiting with abdominal pain)
- At least twice the normal measurements of certain liver enzymes on blood test
- Thrombocytopenia (low platelet count)
- Very low urine output (less than 500 mL in 24 hours)
- Signs of respiratory problems (pulmonary oedema, bluish tint to the skin)
- Severe foetal growth restriction
- Stroke

In this, blood pressure remains a consistent feature. Other criteria may be present one or more in the same woman.

Some publications tend to use the label of moderate pre-eclampsia. In moderate pre-eclampsia, a blood pressure of 140–159 mmHg systolic or 90–159 mmHg diastolic, with no complications of severe pre-eclampsia is included. Proteinuria is again optional.

REFERENCES

1. Brown MA, Magee LA, Kenny LC, Karumanchi SA, McCarthy FP, Saito S, Hall DR, Warren CE, Adoyi G, Ishaku S, International Society for the Study of Hypertension in Pregnancy (ISSHP): The hypertensive disorders of pregnancy: ISSHP classification, diagnosis and management recommendations for international practice. *Pregnancy Hypertens* 13:291–310, 2018. doi:10.1016/j.preghy.2018.05.004. Epub 2018 May 24.
2. Walsh CA, Baxi LV: Mean arterial pressure and prediction of pre-eclampsia. *BMJ* 336(7653):1079–1080, 2008. doi:10.1136/bmj.39555.518750.80.
3. Cnossen JS, Vollebregt KC, de Vrieze N, Ter Riet G, Mol BW, Franx A, Khan KS, et al. Accuracy of mean arterial pressure and

blood pressure measurements in predicting pre-eclampsia: Systematic review and meta-analysis. *BMJ* 336(7653):1117–1120, 2008. doi:10.1136/bmj.39540.522049.BE.

4. Dong X, Gou W, Li C, Wu M, Han Z, Li X, Chen Q: Proteinuria in preeclampsia: Not essential to diagnosis but related to disease severity and fetal outcomes. *Pregnancy Hypertens* 8:60–64, 2017. doi:10.1016/j.preghy.2017.03.005.

5. Shi J, Yang Z, Chen L: Study on the heterogeneity of edema in severe preeclampsia. *Zhonghua Yi Xue Za Zhi* 94(17):1342–1345, 2014 [Article in Chinese].

PART 7

Treatment of pre-eclampsia

16

Treatment of pre-eclampsia

INTRODUCTION

The basic aim of treating pre-eclampsia includes controlling hypertension and preventing complications. In treating hypertension, however, attempting to bring the blood pressure to pre-pregnant level quickly is not desirable. This is important because it can downright harm the mother and the foetus if energetic measures are taken to lower blood pressure. Also, blood pressure will greatly resist attempts to be lowered to pre-pregnancy levels, though the blood pressure may fall transiently. It will, however, spring up while the woman is still pregnant. The ongoing process of pre-eclampsia produces widespread vasospasm in the maternal vasculature. The rise in blood pressure is a reaction to that vasospasm. If through antihypertensives the blood pressure is energetically lowered, the blood flow to the different systems of the gravida and the all-important foetomaternal interface would get seriously reduced, thereby inviting complications.

MANAGEMENT GOALS IN PRE-ECLAMPSIA

Leveno and Cunningham while authoring the chapter on "management of eclampsia" in the book, Chesley's *Hypertensive Disorders of Pregnancy* have concisely defined the basic management goals of a woman with pre-eclampsia.[1] They stated that the basic management objectives for any pregnancy complicated by pre-eclampsia are:

1. Termination of pregnancy with the least possible trauma to the mother or the foetus,

2. Birth of an infant who subsequently thrives and
3. Complete restoration of health to the mother.

These three principles of management are by and large achievable in nearly all women with pre-eclampsia in modern obstetrics. Very elaborate understanding of the aetiopathology and pathophysiology involved, new drugs and the influx of modern technology like colour Doppler in obstetric practice have made it possible.

EARLY DIAGNOSIS AND ALERT SURVEILLANCE

The absolute cut-off value of blood pressure of 130/90 mmHg to label a woman as pre-eclamptic is just one factor. In subjects with antenatal care of a good quality, a more appropriate cut-off level of a rise of 30 mmHg systolic or 15 mmHg diastolic taken on two consecutive readings at least 6 hours apart after adequate bed rest is more accurate. This is more so for petite mothers, especially in the Indian subcontinent and other parts of east Asia. These mothers have a low blood pressure physiologically. Many of these women comfortably maintain their physiology of all organs and systems at blood pressure as low as 90/70 mmHg. There will always be situations that can fool clinicians if they wait for 130/90 mmHg.

One more point that must be considered in alert surveillance is related to the mid-trimester fall in blood pressure registered in normal pregnancy. In women who visit public hospitals in countries like India, the failure of the fall of mid-trimester blood pressure can be missed. This is because these subjects may register late for antenatal care.

133

In such situations, the clinician may not be able to provide the women with the advantages of alert surveillance-based only on this one parameter.

The other aspect where quality surveillance can help is in the late stage of impending eclampsia. An eye on the clinical and laboratory features like worsening proteinuria, rising blood pressure, sudden unusual weight gain, complaints like epigastric pain or dimness of vision and the entire list of features of impending eclampsia greatly helps in quality surveillance. In such women, the termination of pregnancy with the least possible trauma to the mother and the foetus can be planned much before the situation goes out of hand.

DO WOMEN WITH PRE-ECLAMPSIA NEED ADMISSION?

In clinical practice in countries like India, there are two distinct groups of pregnant women: One group of public hospital-class patients who do not have the awareness of the need for antenatal care. The other group is the well-educated and adequately resourced patients who register for antenatal care (usually, in private hospitals and clinics) as early as possible. Expectedly, the outcome in both these group of subjects is bound to be different. As a result, some principles of approach would be a shade different.

Women in whom the importance of antenatal care is not known and their reliability of coming for regular antenatal care cannot be guaranteed, admission for pre-eclampsia, even if mild, may become necessary. However, with the same blood pressure, women in whom adequate follow-up for antenatal care can be ensured, admission may not be necessary at the hospital, and they may be treated at home.

MANAGEMENT ON HOSPITALIZATION

On admission, these women need a systematic management plan. This includes:

- Twice a day measurement of blood pressure.
- Bed rest with restricted activity: By restricted activity it is meant that she can be allowed to go to the toilet for her daily and periodic clean up and wash needs as well as for passing urine and stool. (This is contrasted against "absolute" bed rest where such liberty may not be allowed. Thankfully this is hardly required in modern obstetrics.)
- Testing urine for albuminuria is also to be done every day. An increasing proteinuria may be the first sign of worsening pre-eclampsia. It may indicate a need for an early intervention.
- Biophysical profile: On admission and then after daily, there will be need to perform a biophysical profile of the pregnant woman. Though it may sound too soon, sudden precipitous deteriorations of these subjects can be picked up in this way. It is wise to individualise performing a biophysical assessment in women with severe pre-eclampsia. There can be situations where, if in patient's pre-eclampsia is steadily worsening, there might be a need to perform biophysical profile especially cardiotocography (CTG) tracings even 6 hourly.
- Steroids: Antenatal administration of steroids to improve the foetal systemic maturity, especially the lungs, should be given to the mother; 24 mg of betamethasone administered intramuscularly over an interval of 24–36 hours is the standard schedule.

One controversy that is relevant to the current discussion is to the perception that organ and systemic maturity occurs faster in women with pre-eclampsia. There had been reports and studies, which suggested that babies born to mothers with severe pre-eclampsia and eclampsia have much better systemic maturity when matched for the babies at the same gestational age born to women without pre-eclampsia. They seem to develop respiratory distress syndrome (RDS) and complications like necrotising enterocolitis (NEC) at a much less frequency. Nevertheless, this claim could not be fully substantiated. It was found that this advantage of early maturity of newborns in subjects with pre-eclampsia was not universal. It was only for subjects who had persistent proteinuria along with hypertension. Thus, proteinuria seems to be an important factor in enhanced systemic maturity. Development and persistence of proteinuria indicates a severe form of pre-eclampsia. Because of this, the foetus develops a faster systemic maturity. This may be a natural preparation for the possible early delivery that may occur due to a rapidly developing hostile intrauterine environment.

Besides the administration of steroids to subjects of pre-eclampsia, admitted subjects may also be needed to be subjected periodically to colour Doppler studies. While CTG may be able to give the status of the foetus over a week or so, colour Doppler will give the foetal status at that precise moment. When the results of the two are reviewed in combination, one gets a more accurate idea for decision making regarding the termination of the pregnancy due to developing foetal risk as the pre-eclamptic pregnancy is advancing.

Antihypertensives

Amongst many controversies that are associated with obstetric vasculopathies, one that generates maximum controversy is related to the use of antihypertensives – which antihypertensive is the best, when to use, when not to use and similar controversies take up many pages of any chapter on the treatment of pre-eclampsia. In all such issues, one school of thought is conservative and the other quite contrastingly radical. In such a situation, carefully conducted randomised controlled trials (RCTs) have guided us in making decisions.

DOES MILD PRE-ECLAMPSIA NEED ANTIHYPERTENSIVES?

This question got debated for years. Thankfully an exhaustive review seems to have settled this issue for now. It clearly states that antihypertensive drug therapy for mild to moderate hypertension during pregnancy reduces the risk of severe hypertension. If antihypertensive drugs are to be used, beta-blockers and calcium channel blockers appear to be more effective than the other available options.[2] The original recommendation for not starting antihypertensives in women with mild pre-eclampsia came from results, which showed that foetal outcome in particular and general obstetric outcomes do not alter by starting antihypertensives in such women. However, those recommendations did not become popular in situations where pregnant women may not come for follow-ups regularly or were ill-informed of the dangers of pre-eclampsia. This issue is now settled with the Cochrane review, spelling out the advantage of giving antihypertensives even in mild pre-eclampsia.

CHALLENGES BEFORE TREATING PRE-ECLAMPSIA WITH ANTIHYPERTENSIVES

Any antihypertensive, when considered for use in pregnancy, has to fulfil a few requirements. The primary one is that it should not be teratogenic. In this regard, most antihypertensives in the current domain of physicians are non-teratogenic and, therefore, are safe for use in pregnancy. But angiotensin-converting enzyme (ACE) inhibitors are an exception to this. They are known teratogens. They can cause renal effects if given in the first trimester and can precipitate IUGR or worsen an already existing IUGR later in pregnancy. So if a woman with hypertension is planning a pregnancy and she is on ACE inhibitors, a transition to safer agent should be immediately undertaken before she conceives.

Besides this, the other challenge before putting any antihypertensive to use in pregnancy is its need to be rapidly effective. In this regard, α-methyldopa may be a little "lazy" in generating it full pharmacological effects. Yet this agent is popular with many clinicians and has nothing much against it.

One more challenge before an antihypertensive is to be employed for use in obstetrics is the fact that it should not reduce the blood pressure precipitously. By precipitous reduction, it is meant that it should not be so powerful that blood pressure falls within seconds of its administration and can even be lowered close to hypotensive levels. A classic example in this regard is sodium nitroprusside. This antihypertensive is potent and rapid in action. Its use was primarily confined to women in whom there was an eclamptic fit where there is an urgent need to control her blood pressure. But sodium nitroprusside was found to be precipitous in lowering blood pressure. Such a rapid fall and that to suboptimal levels at times precipitated accidental haemorrhage in pregnant women. It also caused acute foetal distress and even foetal death. Besides these, there is a grave risk of cyanide toxicity and an increase in intracranial pressure as a result of sodium nitroprusside.[3] Apprehensions were expressed regarding nifedipine, one of the most popular calcium channel blockers, that it can precipitously cause a fall in blood pressure. Over a while, this has been disproved and fears allayed.

Some confusion existed regarding how tight hypertension should be controlled in the treatment of pre-eclampsia. This seems to have been settled through a good review.[4] This systematic review set out to compare the effects of "tight" versus "very tight" control of mild to moderate pre-existing or non-proteinuric gestational hypertension on pregnancy outcomes. It found insufficient evidence to determine which degree of control of blood pressure during pregnancy was more effective for improving outcomes for the mother and baby. There was no evidence of a difference between tight and very tight control groups regarding severe pre-eclampsia, induction of labour and caesarean delivery and no cases of eclampsia or maternal deaths.[4] For clinical practice, therefore, the conclusion is that a reasonably good control with blood pressure hovering around 130/80 mmHg could be a good clinical practice.

Another challenge before any antihypertensive are used was to be able to maintain good and effective control over blood pressure during labour. It is well-known that controlling blood pressure can go completely awry during the stress of labour. A violent uterine activity can quickly shunt large amounts of blood from and into the maternal circulation. In such a situation, blood pressure control gets severely challenged and may be lost. A good antihypertensive must be able to control a woman's blood pressure even during this phase.

A challenge that has only recently been met with is the route of antihypertensive administration. Women with eclampsia are unconscious and hypertensive. They can convulse again if the situation is not managed efficiently. Oral administration of antihypertensives in them is nearly impossible. Attempts made by some to administer antihypertensives through the nasogastric tubes were also futile and even dangerous. This is because a convulsive woman may not be able to tolerate the nasogastric tube for long. Also, women with eclampsia have a reduced gastric emptying time. In such a situation, administering anything orally can be vomited out. Vomiting in an unconscious patient is dangerous because it can precipitate Mendelson syndrome. This can be fatal.

For a time, hardly any antihypertensive safe for use in pregnancy parenterally was available. This problem was first solved by the availability of hydralazine. Nifedipine in the meantime was able to solve this problem even before parenteral labetalol became available. Nifedipine could be administered sublingually and so non-oral administration of antihypertensive became a reality even before injectable hydralazine became universally available.

One more challenge that any antihypertensive can face is its mechanism of action. One mechanism by which many antihypertensives act is by reducing the cardiac output. This could be unacceptable to the pregnant woman because it can seriously jeopardize the foetal circulation. In all of these, therefore, agents which reduced peripheral resistance by vasodilatation were found to be most useful. This explains the popularity of nifedipine and hydralazine in PIH as well as eclampsia.

WHICH ANTIHYPERTENSIVE?

This seems to be a perpetual debate and a large volume of research papers have been generated on this. The constant influx of antihypertensives in pharmacological science makes the obstetrician inquisitive if one antihypertensive is better than the other. Thankfully in this matter, the situation is now quite clear. Amongst all antihypertensives that are currently in use, the safest, effective and popular are nifedipine (calcium channel blockers), alpha methyldopa, atenolol and labetalol. Oral nifedipine, and possibly labetalol and methyldopa, are suitable options for treatment of severe hypertension in pregnancy or postpartum.[5] As regards atenolol, it appears to be safe and effective in late pregnancy, while labetalol has an efficacy comparable to methyldopa.[6] It has been proven through a review study that until better evidence is available, the choice of antihypertensive should depend on the clinician's experience and familiarity with a particular drug; on what is known about adverse effects and on women's preferences. Exceptions are nimodipine, magnesium sulphate (although this is indicated for women who require an anticonvulsant for prevention or treatment of eclampsia), diazoxide and ketanserin, which are probably best avoided.[7]

MONO THERAPY VERSUS MULTI-DRUG THERAPY

By and large mono-drug therapy in pre-eclampsia is a rule. Nevertheless, a second drug can be added if blood pressure is not adequately controlled by the highest permissible dose of the single primary drug that is started. It is, therefore, recommended that the dosage of the same drug is increased in a gradient if blood pressure is not controlled. Only if the maximum dose is unable to adequately control the blood pressure, should another drug be added.

For non-oral administration, currently three drugs are available for use: (i) Sublingual nifedipine, (ii) intramuscular labetalol and (iii) intramuscular or intravenous hydralazine.

DRUGS AND THEIR DOSAGE SCHEDULES

Nifedipine

Nifedipine is given in an oral dose of 10 mg every 8 hours. In women with eclampsia or those in whom oral administration is to be restricted, nifedipine is administered in a dose of 5 mg sublingually to be repeated every 6–8 hours. The antihypertensive efficacy of this low-dose nifedipine given sublingually is similar to that of conventional dosage, and the safety profile of low-dose nifedipine dripping pills is better than that of the conventional dose. However, as soon as the pregnant woman can take orally, one can switch over to the oral dosage schedule.

Atenolol

Atenolol is administered in a dose of 25–50 mg/day, initially. If blood pressure is not controlled with this dosage, this can be increased to 100 mg/day. Atenolol usually controls blood pressure using a once-a-day dose. However, if blood pressure is not controlled 25 mg is given every 12 hours until blood pressure is controlled.

Labetalol

Labetalol can be given in a dose of 200 mg every 12 hours to commence with. But as soon as blood pressure is controlled, the dose is reduced to 100 mg every 12 hours.

Alpha methyldopa

Alpha methyldopa is usually started in a dose of 250 mg every 8 hours. However, if this does not suffice to control blood pressure, the dosage can be increased to 250 mg every 6 hours. This can be further increased up to 500 mg every 6 hours. Thus, alpha methyldopa can be given up to 2 g in 24 hours in 4 divided doses.

Hydralazine

Hydralazine is also recommended for use in pregnancy hypertension. It was the only antihypertensive which could be used safely in pregnancy that was available for parenteral administration, especially in the US market. Its recommended dose is an intravenous bolus at a dose of 5–10 mg, depending on the severity of hypertension, and may be administered every 20 minutes up to a maximum dose of 30 mg.

WHEN TO STOP ANTIHYPERTENSIVES

Conventionally practice is that as soon as the diastolic blood pressure drops below 90mmHg or systolic drops below 130 mmHg and the mean arterial pressure below 103, antihypertensives can be stopped safely. However, the problem arises in some women in whom blood pressure suddenly goes to normal immediately after delivery. These are usually women who have a severe form of the condition, including eclampsia. In these subjects, blood pressure can and usually does rise after this so-called "lucid interval". Why blood pressure behaves like this is not exactly known. As regards antihypertensives in such subjects, it is wise to discontinue antihypertensives if blood pressure returns to normal levels even if for a transient duration of time. However, close and periodic monitoring of blood pressure should be continued. As and when blood pressure returns to the levels of hypertension, antihypertensives should be restarted in a graded fashion. By graded fashion, it is meant that a full dose of antihypertensives may not be required in the first instance. It is a matter of wisdom and common sense to administer the drug dose graded to the rise in blood pressure if it starts rising again in pre-eclampsia postpartum.

It is felt that if women with pre-eclampsia register hypertension even after 3 months postpartum it could be a case of chronic hypertension or superimposed pre-eclampsia. It is more so in women in whom pre-pregnancy blood pressure is not known. It is believed that pregnancy may reveal hidden hypertension in some. The crux of the matter is that if any woman registers hypertension that needs antihypertensives even after 3 months postpartum, it is wise to seek an opinion of a physician and start investigating and treating these women as a chronic hypertensive.

Having managed the hypertension of a subject with PIH, the next critical decision making for the clinician is the induction of labour.

Induction of labour in PIH

Labour induction can be indicated in many varied clinical situations in pre-eclampsia. The easiest answer is at 37 completed weeks of pregnancy.

But this answer may not necessarily be as simple as it may appear. This is because the decision making is dependent on the severity of the disease, the condition of the unborn child and the maternal complications that may or may not have occurred.

37 WEEKS

37 weeks of pregnancy as a cut-off limit for intervention is accepted following many studies, the latest being one by Fiolna et al.[8] This is with the basis that at this duration of pregnancy, the foetus is matured enough to survive the extra-uterine environment. Once the foetus achieves the systemic maturity, all it has to gain now in the uterus is in weight at the rate of about 23 g/day. Maternal systems confer both the maturity as well as weight to the growing foetus. Most of the challenges that prematurely newborns encounter are essentially due to a deficient maturity. This precipitates life-threatening problems like RDS, NEC and generalised infections including septicaemia. In subjects of PIH in particular, especially severe PIH, if 37 weeks of pregnancy has already been achieved, labour should be induced. However, the bigger challenge lies in subjects who have not yet reached 37 weeks and labour for various reasons needs to be induced. It will be a more challenging decision-making exercise.

INDUCTION OF LABOUR IN ECLAMPSIA

This is one easier decision-making situation. By and large, in most of the pregnant women, once a convulsion following PIH occurs, it is wise to induce labour. The concept of intercurrent eclampsia waxes and wanes in time. There are times when some enthusiasts start advocating controlling the convulsions, preventing subsequent convulsions and allowing the pregnancy to continue. This is intercurrent eclampsia. It is argued that if the pregnancy has not yet reached a stage where neonatal survival chances are good, such pregnancies are continued beyond the convulsion. Most believe that allowing the maternal system to bear the fierce onslaught of hypertension in its most severe form is unnecessary and unjustified. We do not believe in the concept of intercurrent eclampsia. We induce labour in any subject of eclampsia irrespective of the duration of pregnancy. We only wait for a few hours of a convulsion maximum two for the convulsing mother to settle and then initiate measures of inducing labour.

INDUCTION OF LABOUR IN SEVERE PRE-ECLAMPSIA

Having had seen the two relatively easy indications for labour induction, now some tougher areas need to be reviewed. One such area is severe PIH. There are some groups of research workers who clump severe PIH and imminent eclampsia together. Therefore, in their subjects, severe hypertension characterised by blood pressure at or above 110 mmHg diastolic and proteinuria of >1 g/day are principle factors deciding in favour of induction of labour. These may be coupled by minor factors like sudden severe weight gain, oliguria, epigastric pain, persistent headache or visual alterations, and the like. This bunch of features is considered minor and therefore, contributes to decision making. But in themselves, they do not clinch the issue on their own.

INDUCTION OF LABOUR IN PREGNANCY FOR FOETAL REASONS

In these subjects, the need for induction arises purely because the unborn foetus is developing features of compromise, including IUGR. The other feature that may be accompanying IUGR is oligohydramnios. Thus, IUGR and oligohydramnios singly or in combination are an indication for labour induction in subjects of PIH. This is the toughest decision-making situation. In this, blood pressure has still not crossed the limits to be labelled as severe PIH. Also, there are no life-threatening complications for the mother. To make matters worse for decision making, the pregnancy has still not reached the comfort zone of 37 weeks and beyond. These are the pregnancies where decision making is the toughest. However, the toughest part is to decide when to induce labour in such a pregnancy. It is, therefore, rightly said that when the intrauterine environment is more hostile for the foetus as compared to the extra-uterine environment, the pregnancy needs to be terminated. Having had understood this principle, now the challenge lies in deciding and correctly diagnosing this hostility of the environment.

For this purpose, clinical as well as technological inputs and their correlation become critical. Relying solely on any one of the two could invite a grave possibility of iatrogenic prematurity, which is completely preventable and understandably unnecessary. As regards the clinical diagnosis, it is based on parameters like a symphysis-fundal height (SFH). If the pregnancy has a difference of 6 cm or more of SFH at or after 30 weeks of pregnancy, IUGR or oligohydramnios should be suspected. This method has its limitations of reliability but is often the first sign alerting the clinician.

Even a regular antenatal check-up can alert the clinician to a possibility of the baby not thriving within. This needs just an average experience and no extraordinary expertise. Most clinicians have done away with the practice of measuring the SFM. In such a situation, even regular alert palpation of the fundus and assessing its height with context to the weeks of gestation as per the menstrual age is sufficient for the same.

The other vital help that is received is from colour Doppler and CTG tracings. These two have been extensively discussed elsewhere. Based on ultrasonography, oligohydramnios is diagnosed easily. Also, ultrasonography will help in diagnosing a head-sparing type of IUGR by automatically plotting the ratio of head circumference to the abdominal circumference. If this is increasing (even if within the normal range), it will be diagnosed as IUGR and alert the clinician to a possible need for early intervention. Besides the head circumference-to-abdominal circumference (HC/AC) ratio and amniotic fluid index (AFI), serial ultrasound will also show a decline in expected birth weight (EBW). When plotted on a graph, this decline is so obvious that it cannot be missed.

One important marker for identifying a reduced foetal growth rate is cerebroplacental ratio (CPR) of the umbilical artery at or near term on colour Doppler. Studies have shown that the CPR is a marker of impaired foetal growth velocity and adverse pregnancy outcome, even in foetuses whose size is considered appropriate using conventional biometry.[9] The basis of this ratio is that the foetal system when healthy maintains the blood supply and oxygenation with a bias towards the brain. As a result, the pulsatility index of the brain is more than that of the umbilical artery.

In numerical terms, this ratio will be ≥ 1. However, when the ratio is ≤ 1, it suggests that the foetus is hypoxic and endangered. As a result, it warrants immediate intervention. Thus, in such women, induction may be indicated even if pre-eclampsia has not worsened.

On the other hand, this ratio is so sensitive that a pregnancy can be prolonged if the CPR is maintained above 1. This is shown in the following case study.

CASE STUDY IN CPR

Mrs. S, 29 years G_6P_3, was referred to us as having oligoamnios at 27 weeks of pregnancy. This oligoamnios was of placental origin as foetal origin was ruled out through targeted scan for foetal malformations.

Her Obstetric History strongly indicated a perpetual process of obstetric vasculopathy:

- First two foetal demise at 28–30 weeks, both instances PIH and IUGR.
- The third was a spontaneous demise at 11 weeks after fetal heart activity was seen.
- Fourth was a full-term stillbirth severe PIH with IUGR.

AFI was as shown in Figure 16.1. The condition of the foetus was obviously compromised as shown in the graphs in Figure 16.2. The EFW was below the standard deviation and the AFI was low. The foetus not only had oligoamnios but also IUGR. This indicated that this time also the process of obstetric vasculopathy was in full swing. The question now was whether to deliver as a knee-jerk response or wait. To wait, she needed colour Doppler for assuring the safety of the foetus in the intrauterine environment. Her colour Doppler of middle cerebral artery (MCA) was as shown in Figure 16.3. Colour Doppler of the umbilical artery was as shown in Figure 16.4. From Figures 16.3 and 16.4, the CPR was 1.34. This was above 1 and so the pregnancy was continued. She was already on aspirin 75 mg/day, which was continued. She was put on a weekly follow-up. Her CPR remained above 1. At 33 weeks 4 days, her baby continued to have IUGR with low-normal AFI, as shown in Figure 16.5. The EFW was 1876 g. Her MCA showed a PI (Pulsatility Index) of 1.38, as shown in Figure 16.6. Her umbilical artery PI at this stage was 1, as shown in Figure 16.7. CPR calculated

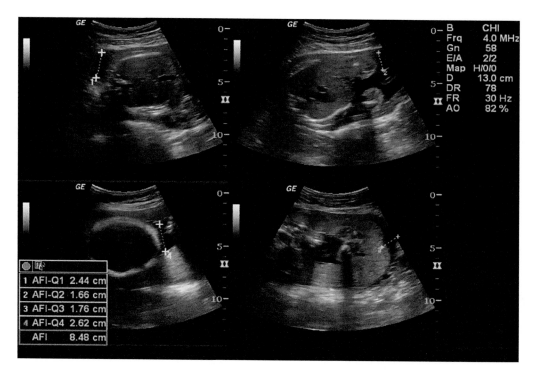

Figure 16.1 Amniotic fluid index at 27 weeks.

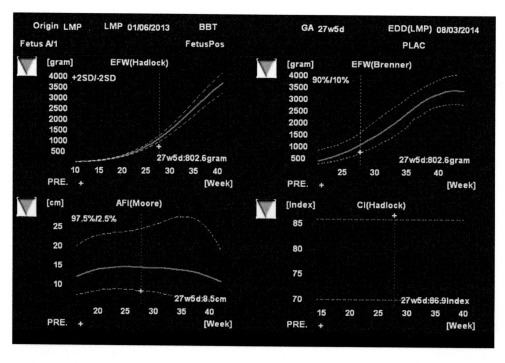

Figure 16.2 Graphs at 27 weeks.

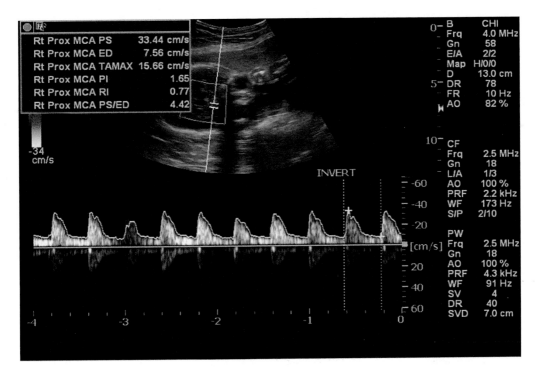

Figure 16.3 Indices of middle cerebral artery (MCA) flow at 27 weeks.

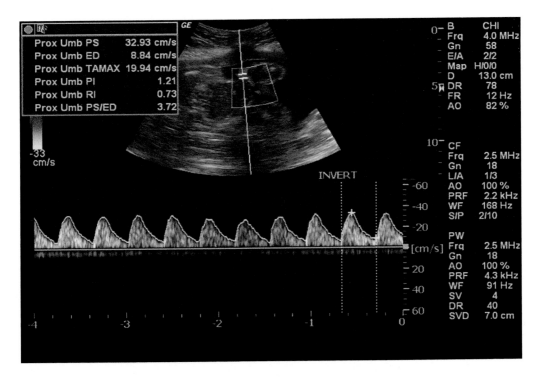

Figure 16.4 Indices of umbilical artery flow at 27 weeks.

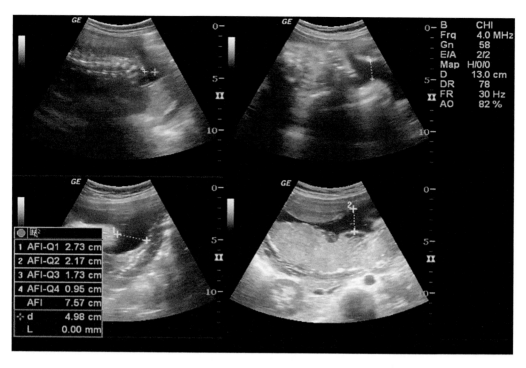

Figure 16.5 Amniotic fluid index at 33 weeks.

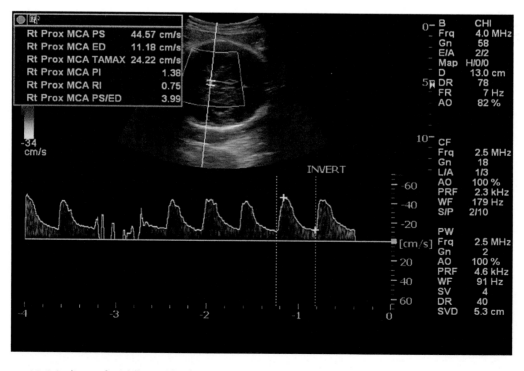

Figure 16.6 Indices of middle cerebral artery (MCA) flow at 33 weeks.

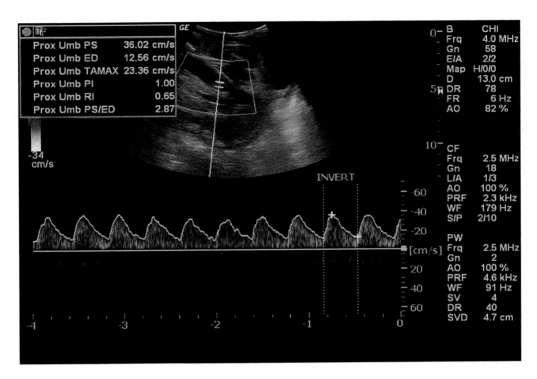

Prox Umb PS	36.02 cm/s
Prox Umb ED	12.56 cm/s
Prox Umb TAMAX	23.36 cm/s
Prox Umb PI	1.00
Prox Umb RI	0.65
Prox Umb PS/ED	2.87

Figure 16.7 Indices of umbilical artery flow at 33 weeks.

thus came to 1.38. Therefore, we waited. At 37 weeks, her blood pressure shot up to 160/100 mmHg. Obstetric intervention was done, and she delivered a full-term IUGR newborn of 2060 g. Both, the mother as well as the newborn was well.

Analysis of the case study

This case study is representative of the competence of CPR in identifying the foetal well-being in the intrauterine environment. This pregnancy, which was on the threshold of getting induced merely based on liquor and IUGR could be carried to full term. Until that time as the brain of the foetus continues to receive a preference in circulation as reflected by the pulsatility index of the MCA being greater than that of the umbilical artery, the foetus is safe in the intrauterine environment. Foetal CPR is predictive of caesarean section for intrapartum foetal compromise, small for gestational age and foetal growth restriction and neonatal intensive care unit (NICU) admission. Low CPR can also be significantly associated with abnormal foetal heart rate pattern, meconium-stained liquor,

low Apgar score, acidosis at birth and composite adverse perinatal outcome scores. The CPR, when taken at term, had comparable if not better predictive value than that when taken at preterm.[10]

Until that time, as the utility of CPR as a standalone marker for predicting the foetal condition in utero is established, there is a need to use other markers in this process. One such is CTG. Once the clinician is alerted to the possibility of the baby suffering from chronic hypoxia, the vital decision making that is required relates to if and when to deliver the baby. In this situation, colour Doppler and CTG together help significantly.

The CTG analyses the behaviour of foetal heart rate and rhythm gives an idea of foetal oxygenation status over a small period of time. Any significant alteration in the variability of the foetal heart rate and rhythm is ominous. Also if the foetal heart rate refuses to accelerate with foetal movement, it is ominous. If during the course of evaluation, the foetal heart rate registers a deceleration on a non-stress test (NST), it is ominous. Any one or more of these features indicate that the foetus is in trouble and needs to be delivered.

These three technological inputs showed that the intrauterine environment was hostile for the foetus, and therefore, it was wise to induce labour. So, in the clinical situation of a pregnancy being less than 37 weeks, and if the decision making about induction of labour is necessitated, it is the most difficult of all indications of induction labour in PIH.

THE NEED FOR INVOLVING A NEONATOLOGIST

As a part of improved antenatal care and quality obstetrics, it is now a rule in all good obstetric units to involve the neonatologist in decision making about induction of labour in difficult situations. There are important inputs, which are obtained from the neonatologist, the main being how early or preterm child will the neonatal unit be able to handle. In this context, most good units are now reasonably confident in handling the average birth weight of 1,000 g or more. Many of these units are salvaging babies as small as 700 g in weight and about 26 weeks in maturity. However, with better technology, ventilator support and the availability of surfactants, still younger and lighter babies will be salvaged.

The second reason to involve a neonatologist in this decision making is to help the unit get prepared for handling of such a baby. Gone are the days when obstetricians used to operate in isolation. It is no more only their concern when to induce labour. Working in isolation can open up scenarios where an unprepared and overloaded NICU unit receives a sick baby it is unable to take in or optimally handle. It is, therefore, necessary to involve the neonatologist in decision making regarding the timing of induction in pregnancies less than 37 weeks in duration

READINESS OF THE MATERNAL SYSTEM FOR LABOUR INDUCTION IN PIH

It is interesting to note that the maternal system is many times ready to get labour induction going in situations of severe PIH and eclampsia. This is attributed to the process of decidual activation that is the key harbinger of labour. With the understanding of the physiology of labour becoming more and more clear, it has become obvious that labour is induced not by the mother but by the foetal systems. If the intrauterine environment is non-conducive to pregnancy continuation, labour gets induced much more easily. This does not need the foetus to be alive. Even if the foetus has had a demise, labour gets readily induced to eliminate the product of conception.

The concept of the foetal unit having a key and decisive role in inducing labour came from the observation that foetuses with anencephaly in pre-ultrasound days could not be diagnosed so easily. As a result, labour induction in anencephalic foetus would not happen readily. The anencephalic foetus was a known cause of postdatism in those days. Hence, a challenged and endangered foetal system in obstetric vasculopathy supports attempts at labour induction readily.

METHODS OF THE INDUCTION OF LABOUR

Use of prostaglandins has made induction of labour easier, more controlled and less arduous. In reality, prostaglandins are so easily available for the purpose that now the onus is on the obstetrician to ensure that it is not misused or overused. Also, the safety profile becomes a matter of concern with this relatively new pharmacological technology.

Trachleodynamics in the induction of labour

While on methods of inducing labour, it is necessary to understand the cervix, its dynamics, and physiology for successful and safe labour induction. The cervix needs to be evaluated for its favourability for labour induction. In this context, Bishop's score has been of great help in clinical practice for decades now. The Bishop score (also known as pelvic score) is the most commonly used method to judge the readiness of the cervix for induction of labour. The Bishop score gives points to five measurements of the pelvic examination dilation, effacement of the cervix, station of the foetus, consistency of the cervix and position of the cervix. Bishop score was subsequently modified by Calder has been now well established. Some studies did express the reservations about

Table 16.1 Bishop score for induction of labour

Parameter\Score	0	1	2	3
Position	Posterior	Intermediate	Anterior	–
Consistency	Firm	Intermediate	Soft	–
Effacement	0%–30%	31%–50%	51%–80%	>80%
Dilation	0 cm	1–2 cm	3–4 cm	>5 cm
Foetal station	−3	−2	−1, 0	+1, +2

the competence of Bishop score.[11] Nevertheless, its popularity remains unaffected (Table 16.1).

A score of more than 6 indicates a favourable cervix for induction of labour and will result in a successful outcome more after than not.

The concept of trachleodynamics needs to be carefully understood in subjects with obstetric vasculopathies, including PIH. This is so because on more occasions than not, labour inducing interventions need to be employed. For the success of any labour induction, cervical compliance and subsequent synchronous dilatation have to happen. Cervical ripening agents are expected to bring about a series of changes in the ultrastructure and biochemical milieu in such a way that cervix becomes shortened, softened and dilated to let the passage of the foetus. This transforms the cervix from a sphincter organ, which preserves the pregnancy to a dilated conduit letting the foetus pass through it. In this process, prostaglandins have proven to be the "game changers".

Before the introduction of prostaglandins in the induction of labour, most pharmacological agents like oxytocin used to act on the uterus. Their uterine predominance activated the activity in the uterus secondary to which the cervix dilated. However, in the physiology of labour, this is not the way labour initiates and progresses. In physiology, the cervix becomes compliant, softens and dilates proactively. The uterine activity is occurring in symphony with the cervical ripening and dilatation in rhythm. None is secondary to the other. As a result, drugs and methods that envisaged inducing labour by bringing about uterine activity and letting the cervix respond secondarily to the uterus take a long time for labour to get induced. Often, these methods fail. They also tended to need other ancillary measures to activate the process. These include methods like stripping of membranes or artificial rupture of membranes.

Prostaglandins

Both prostaglandins, PGE2 and PGF2α, are used to activate cervix and induce labour in PIH. However, PGE2 is predominantly active on the cervix. Therefore, their action is more useful for cervical softening and ripening. PGF2α seems to be more selective for uterus in its action, though it too has a weak direct action on the cervix. Therefore, PGE2 is used predominantly for labour induction by cervical ripening.

When oral and vaginal prostaglandins were compared, oral PG was less effective than vaginal PG gel in achieving vaginal birth in less than 24 h. However, oral PG was safer because it resulted in fewer CS (Cesarean Sections) without increasing maternal morbidity or neonatal asphyxia.[12] However, there is a small disadvantage of possible hyperstimulation of the uterus. There is an unresolved inconsistency observed for the hyperstimulation outcome following the use of prostaglandins in labour induction.[13] Over a while, with obstetricians becoming more and more used to prostaglandin use, hyperstimulation is no more menacing and widespread. Carefully graded doses of administration of prostaglandins have nearly eliminated the fear of uterine rupture.

DOSE

Intracervical PGF2α gels are available as 0.5 and 1 mg dispensation for cervical ripening. In subjects of PIH with an unripe cervix (Bishop score <4), it is recommended to start with a dose of 1 mg of intracervical or vaginal gel. This is to be repeated every 6 hours for a maximum of a total dose of 4 mg in 24 hours. This dose may be reduced for multigravida proportionately. In multigravida, the maximum dose recommended is 3 mg in 24 hours.

It is wise to monitor the uterine activity for the initial half an hour to 1 hour of PGE2 gel administration for diagnosing uterine hyperstimulation secondary to which there can also be foetal distress. Currently, PGE2 is also administered in a dose of 0.5 mg initially as cervical or vaginal gel followed by 0.5 mg every 6 hours. This has nearly eliminated the fear of uterine hyperstimulation and consequent foetal distress. A good review has reported that PGE2 probably increases the chance of vaginal delivery in 24 hours; they also increase uterine hyperstimulation with foetal heart changes but do not affect or may reduce caesarean section rates. They increase the likelihood of cervical change, with no increase in operative delivery rates. PGE2 tablets, gels and pessaries appear to be as effective as each other, and any differences between formulations are marginal.[14]

Once the cervix becomes ripe and Bishop score is >6, it is advised to administer PGF2α vaginally in a dose of 25 μg per vaginum. This is given every 4–6 hours. PGF2α has its predominant uterine action. This action coupled with a compliant cervix creates a completely physiological situation for proper and successful labour induction. Most of the times, labour with these doses get induced within 24 hours successfully.

Foley catheters in induction of labour

There are a few mechanical methods for inducing labour. This includes artificial rupture of membranes and stripping of membranes. Amongst all these, Foley catheter balloons are the most commonly used mechanical device for labour induction currently. It acts both as a mechanical dilator of the cervix as well as a stimulator of prostaglandins released from the foetal membranes. Compared with vaginal PGE2 gel in term labour induction, a Foley catheter achieved similar vaginal delivery rates, with fewer maternal and neonatal side effects.[15] A Foley catheter left in place for up to 12 hours brings about cervical changes sufficient for term labour induction, and shorter ripening time is associated with earlier artificial rupture of the membranes and start of oxytocin augmentation, which might be related to quicker labour onset.[16] In this, the cervix is visualised by a speculum examination, and the catheter is passed feeling that the balloon is between the amniotic sac and the lower uterine segment. The balloon is then inflated with about 30 mL of saline solution and left in place. For women with an unfavourable cervix at term, including those with pre-eclampsia, induction of labour with a Foley catheter is safe and effective. Higher balloon volume (80 mL vs 30 mL) and longer ripening time (24 hours vs 12 hours) would not shorten the induction to delivery interval or reduce caesarean section rate.[16]

Other methods of labour induction

Before prostaglandins got established in this indication, the principle pharmacological agent that was used was oxytocin. Other than pharmacological agents, mechanical agents were also used in the process. These included hygroscopic cervical dilators, balloon catheters and the like. These were met with reasonable success but did not become popular.

Another set of mechanical methods of labour induction included milieu-altering methods. These were methods probably to induce labour by disturbing the stable environment of an ongoing pregnancy. These include membrane stripping and artificial rupture of membranes. These met with inconsistent success. Besides, their popularity was only because better methods were not available. There was always a grave risk of chorioamnionitis. If after an artificial rupture of membranes, labour failed to get induced within a reasonable time (24 hours), there was a real risk of chorioamnionitis. This could prove fatal both for the foetus and the mother. As soon as prostaglandins became available for labour induction, these methods quickly fell by the wayside.

Once labour got induced, the progress monitoring in PIH is always more vigilant. This is because a compromised foetus would get distressed much earlier compared to low-risk pregnancy foetuses. Continuous CTG monitoring in labour is not out of place. Caesarean section incidence is, therefore, likely to be higher in subjects of severe PIH.

CAESAREAN SECTION IN PIH

The whens, whys and hows of caesarean section in PIH is an interesting aspect of obstetric management. Though caesarean section rates may be little higher in subjects with severe PIH, this is not an absolute indication. The only absolute indication for caesarean section in pre-eclampsia and eclampsia is status eclampticus. Needless to say, obstetric indications of caesarean section like cephalopelvic disproportion, mentoposterior and the like will warrant a caesarean section irrespective of pre-eclampsia.

Caesarean section for PIH is a much more complicated and challenging issue, which needs the fundamentals to be understood. If one revisits indication for doing lower segment caesarean section (LSCS) purely for PIH, then the list is short with either one or two entries. The most common amongst all is when PIH gets complicated with IUGR. In such cases, if CTG and colour Doppler indicate a rapid intervention, the obstetrician may need to carry out a caesarean section.

Rarer amongst the two is a situation where severe PIH continues to worsen despite antihypertensives and other concurrent treatments. If blood pressure is not controlled with or without systemic complications like a renal compromise or coagulation failure, then there is a need for quick intervention to end the pregnancy. This is debatable and thankfully rare. However, in an above-average clinical practice load, obstetricians will have some subjects like these periodically, wherein in view of a rapidly developing situation, caesarean section may be carried out. However, it would always be wise to individualise decision making. Except for these two, there is hardly any situation where PIH may need a caesarean section.

POST-DELIVERY CARE

The final management comes in related to post-delivery management.

Postpartum haemorrhage (PPH)

Once the woman has delivered, there are a series of problems that need to be watchfully dealt by a clinician. The biggest dread is a possibility of PPH. For reasons still not amply clear, subjects with severe PIH tend to develop atonic PPH. This is a tricky situation to handle. Methyl ergometrine, the known strong uterotonic, is notorious for elevating blood pressure. In women with PIH, one can ill afford this situation. It would, therefore, be a challenge to the dexterity of a clinician to weigh between administration of methyl ergometrine for prevention and treatment of atonic PPH in women with PIH on one side and handling a sudden elevation of blood pressure on the other.

Usually, methyl ergometrine is avoided for preventing of atonic PPH in severe PIH. Instead, milder agents like syntocinon are administered. However, when and if atonic PPH occurs, the clinician does take a calculated risk and administers methyl ergometrine. At that moment, the critical decision is to weigh between allowing a potentially fatal blood loss and managing a fresh rise in blood pressure. The decision usually goes in favour of stopping blood loss. The rise in blood pressure is usually handled by sublingual nifedipine or parenteral labetalol. Many clinicians prefer the use of prostaglandins like $PGF2\alpha$ for prevention of PPH in subjects with pre-eclampsia.

Blood pressure

Irrespective of PPH, sometimes blood pressure tends to behave erratically postpartum. In most subjects, blood pressure gradually falls in a graded pattern and returns to pre-pregnant levels by the time puerperium ends. Accordingly, the clinician will be required to taper the dose of antihypertensives. Nevertheless, there will be some subjects in whom blood pressure can suddenly appear normotensive in the early puerperium about 48 hours post-delivery. But it can then catapult to the high pre-delivery levels quickly then after. For a clinician, it is necessary to be aware of the dose adjustments of antihypertensives that will be required. It is possible that in the phase in which the blood pressure suddenly falls to "normal" levels immediately postpartum, it may necessitate a complete withdrawal of antihypertensives. Then afterwards, the antihypertensives may need to be reintroduced if blood pressure starts to rise again.

Coagulation failure

Severe PIH can be complicated by a relatively rare complication of coagulation failure in the postpartum phase. This process starts just when the process is at its peak before delivery but may get menacingly manifested as PPH. Replacement of coagulation factors in the form of whole fresh blood or blood components is the established form of treatment. However, it can severely challenge an already precariously balanced system.

Renal failure

This complication of PIH also becomes manifested most of the times postpartum. A precariously balanced renal function gets ticked off with the added load of blood loss in subjects of PIH. Consequently, there renal failure can be clinically manifested in such conditions. Thankfully these are most of the times glomerular failure. However, if a cortical failure occurs, it can be difficult to reverse. The subject may need dialysis and renal transplantation.

It is noteworthy that the effect of PPH resulting in renal failure occurs much more readily in subjects with pre-eclampsia or eclampsia. This vulnerability arises from the reversal of physiology in hypertensive disorders of pregnancy. The increase in blood volume that occurs in pregnancy as a part of physiological adaptation can be as high as 1.5 L by term. In PIH, this increase in blood volume is either completely or partially curtailed. As a result, the maternal systems work on low circulating blood volume. Consequently, renal failure can occur with relative ease in women with pre-eclampsia. An impoverished renal system of blood volume and sick kidneys innate to PIH precipitates renal shut down readily. The PPH in pre-eclampsia also occurs readily with relatively less blood loss as compared to blood loss in women without pre-eclampsia. As a result, women with pre-eclampsia are more vulnerable to these complications in the postpartum period.

Pulmonary oedema

One more complication that a clinician needs to be watchful about while managing the puerperium of a woman with pre-eclampsia is pulmonary oedema. Fluid imbalance can also readily occur in the postpartum period of women with pre-eclampsia. This is due to two reasons:

1. The extracellular fluid that had increased (manifesting clinically as oedema) now starts reversing in the postpartum period.
2. The process of hypertension itself makes the woman vulnerable to this imbalance.

In such a delicately balanced scenario, if the clinician is not careful in administering fluids, the cardiovascular system can get readily off balance, producing pulmonary oedema. It would, therefore, be a challenge for the clinician to have a sound understanding of the pathophysiology of hypertensive disorders of pregnancy to dexterously manage the woman puerperium.

REFERENCES

1. Leveno K, Cunningham G: In Lindheimer M, Roberts J, Cunningham F, editors: *Chesley, Hypertensive Disorders of Pregnancy*, 2nd ed., p. 547, 1998, Stamford, CT, Appleton & Lange.
2. Abalos E, Duley L, Steyn DW, Gialdini C: Antihypertensive drug therapy for mild to moderate hypertension during pregnancy. *Cochrane Database Syst Rev* (10):CD002252, 2018. doi:10.1002/14651858.CD002252.pub4.
3. McCoy S, Baldwin K: Pharmacotherapeutic options for the treatment of preeclampsia. *Am J Health Syst Pharm* 66(4):337–344, 2009. doi:10.2146/ajhp080104.
4. Nabhan AF, Elsedawy MM: Tight control of mild-moderate pre-existing or non-proteinuric gestational hypertension. *Cochrane Database Syst Rev* (7):CD006907, 2011. doi:10.1002/14651858.CD006907.pub2.
5. Firoz T, Magee LA, MacDonell K, Payne BA, Gordon R, Vidler M, von Dadelszen P, Community Level Interventions for Pre-eclampsia (CLIP) Working Group: Oral antihypertensive therapy for severe hypertension in pregnancy and postpartum: A systematic review. *BJOG* 121(10):1210–1218, discussion 1220, 2014. doi:10.1111/1471-0528.12737. Epub 2014 May 16.
6. Kintiraki E, Papakatsika S, Kotronis G, Goulis DG, Kotsis V: Pregnancy-induced hypertension. *Hormones (Athens)* 14(2):211–223, 2015. doi:10.14310/horm.2002.1582.
7. Duley L, Meher S, Jones L: Drugs for treatment of very high blood pressure during pregnancy. *Cochrane Database Syst Rev* (7):CD001449, 2013. doi:10.1002/14651858.CD001449.pub3.

8. Fiolna M, Kostiv V, Anthoulakis C, Akolekar R, Nicolaides KH: Prediction of adverse perinatal outcome by cerebroplacental ratio in women undergoing induction of labor. *Ultrasound Obstet Gynecol* 53(4):473–480, 2019. doi:10.1002/uog.20173. Epub 2019 Mar 4.

9. Khalil A, Morales-Rosello J, Khan N, Nath M, Agarwal P, Bhide A, Papageorghiou A, Thilaganathan B: Is cerebroplacental ratio a marker of impaired fetal growth velocity and adverse pregnancy outcome? *Am J Obstet Gynecol* 216(6):606.e1–606.e10, 2017. doi:10.1016/j.ajog.2017.02.005. Epub 2017 Feb 8.

10. Dunn L, Sherrell H, Kumar S: Review: Systematic review of the utility of the fetal cerebroplacental ratio measured at term for the prediction of adverse perinatal outcome. *Placenta* 54:68–75, 2017. doi:10.1016/j.placenta.2017.02.006. Epub 2017 Feb 12.

11. Kolkman DG, Verhoeven CJ, Brinkhorst SJ, van der Post JA, Pajkrt E, Opmeer BC, Mol BW: The Bishop's score as a predictor of labor induction success: A systematic review. *Am J Perinatol* 30(8):625–630, 2013. doi:10.1055/s-0032-1331024. Epub 2013 Jan 2.

12. Thorbiörnson A, Vladic T, Stjernholm YV: Oral versus vaginal prostaglandin for labor induction. *J Matern Fetal Neonatal Med* 30(7):789–792, 2017. doi:10.1080/14767058.2016.1190823. Epub 2016 Jun 13.

13. Alfirevic Z, Keeney E, Dowswell T, Welton NJ, Dias S, Jones LV, Navaratnam K, Caldwell DM: Labour induction with prostaglandins: A systematic review and network meta-analysis. *BMJ* 350:h217, 2015. doi:10.1136/bmj.h217.

14. Thomas J, Fairclough A, Kavanagh J, Kelly AJ: Vaginal prostaglandin (PGE2 and PGF2a) for induction of labour at term. *Cochrane Database Syst Rev* (6):CD003101, 2014. doi:10.1002/14651858.CD003101.pub3.

15. Jozwiak M, Oude Rengerink K, Benthem M, van Beek E, Dijksterhuis MG, de Graaf IM, vanHuizen ME et al.: In PROBAAT study group. Foley catheter versus vaginal prostaglandin E2 gel for induction of labour at term (PROBAAT trial): An open-label, randomised controlled trial. *Lancet* 378(9809):2095–2103, 2011.

16. Gu N, Ru T, Wang Z, Dai Y, Zheng M, Xu B, Hu Y: Foley catheter for induction of labor at term: An open-label, randomized controlled trial. *PLoS One* 10(8):e0136856, 2015. doi:10.1371/journal.pone.0136856. Published 2015 Aug 31.

Index

Note: Page numbers in italic and bold refer to figures and tables, respectively.

A

AAT (alpha-1 antitrypsin), 39
ACE I/D (angiotensin-converting
 enzyme insertion/
 deletion), 27
aetiology, *58*
alpha-1 antitrypsin (AAT), 39
alpha methyldopa, 137
amniotic fluid index (AFI), 139,
 140, *142*
angiotensin-converting enzyme
 insertion/deletion (ACE
 I/D), 27
antenatal care importance, 134
antihypertensives, 86, 135
 challenges, 135–136
 lucid interval, 137
 mild pre-eclampsia need, 135
 mono therapy *versus* multi-drug
 therapy, 136–137
antiphospholipid antibodies, 17–18
areol, 11
arteries/arterioles, *15*
aspirin, 87
 action, 87–88
 dose of, 88–89
 literature review, 88
 misgivings and fears, 89
 pre-eclampsia, 87
 timing, 89
atenolol, 137
autonomous tight unit, 10

B

balanced atom, *24*
basal metabolic rate (BMR), 52–53
β-hCG, 70
Bishop score, 144, **145**
blood pressure, *52*, 147
BMR (basal metabolic rate), 52–53
body mass index (BMI), 67
brain, 96

C

caesarean section in PIH, 146–147
calcium supplementation, 86–87
calcium-to-creatinine ratio, 68
capillary wall, *16*
carbohydrates, 53
cardiac functions, 99, *100*
cardiac output
 heart increase, 99
 vascular response, 100
cardiotocography (CTG), 143
carotid circulation and block, *36*
cellular components, 68–70
 blood, 20, 103–104
central nervous system (CNS), 95
cerebroplacental ratio (CPR)
 analysis, 143–144
 case study in, 139–143
cervical intraepithelial neoplasia
 (CIN), 84
chronic hypertension, 127

CIN (cervical intraepithelial
 neoplasia), 84
clinical manifestations, 35
clinical tests, 66–67
CNS (central nervous system), 95
coagulation alterations, 104
coagulation factors, 103
coagulation failure, 147
colour Doppler, 71
 and biomarker, 73–74
 diastolic notch, 72–73, *73*
 for discontinuation, 75
 first trimester, low-risk subjects
 in, 76
 indices review, 71–72
 indices with biomarkers, 72
 NDI, 74–75, *75*
CPR, *see* cerebroplacental ratio
 (CPR)
crosstalk, 12
CTG (cardiotocography), 143
cyclooxygenase, 33
cytokines, 19
cytotrophoblasts, 10

D

deadly quartet, 51
derangements, 83
diastolic notch, 72–73, *73*
disease *versus* derangement, 83–84
diuretics, 85–86

Doppler indices, biomarkers, 72
double-edged sword, 24

E

ECE (endothelin converting
    enzyme), 19
ecNOS (endothelial constitutive
    nitric oxide synthase), 41
electrons, 23
endothelial activation
    circulating markers, 16
    prostaglandins, 16–17
endothelial cell activation
    molecules contributing to, 19–20
    phenomenon, 16
    plasminogen and allied
        procoagulant activity, 17
endothelial cell adhesion molecule
    disturbances, 18
    clinical bearings, 18–19
    VWF, 18
endothelial cells, 41–42
endothelial constitutive nitric oxide
    synthase (ecNOS), 41
endothelin, 19
Endothelin-1 (ET-1), 19
endothelin converting enzyme
    (ECE), 19
endothelium, 15
epidemiological indices, 70–71
epigenetics, 61
examining associations, 59
exosomes, xi, 76–77
extracellular reducing systems,
    42–43
extracellular vesicle, 76

F

Fetal Medicine Foundation
    (FMF), 89
fibronectin, 18, 70
focal segmental glomerular
    sclerosis (FSGS), 121
foetal contributions, 59–60
foetomaternal interface, 25
free radical, 23–24, *24*
    family of, 38
    in vascular walls, 25

G

genetic models application, 59
genome-wide association studies, 57
gestational diabetes mellitus
    (GDM), 53
gestational hypertension, 127
ghost ovum, 60
glomeruli, 119–120
glutathione peroxides, 33
gross changes in kidneys, 119

H

haematological indices, 68
haemochorial, 11
haemolysis, elevated liver enzymes,
    low platelet count
    (HELLP) syndrome, 27,
    58, 110, 118–119
hand-grip test, 67
HDL (high-density lipoprotein),
    26, *26*
HELLP (haemolysis, elevated liver
    enzymes, low platelet
    count) syndrome, 27, 58,
    110, 118–119
hepatobiliary system, 109–110
HIF (Hypoxia Inducible Factor), 39
high-density lipoprotein (HDL),
    26, *26*
histotroph, 11
hydralazine, 137
hydroxyl radical, *34*
hypertension, 127–128
hypertriglyceridemia, 31
Hypoxia Inducible Factor (HIF), 39
hypoxic environment, 39

I

ideal reducing systems, 45
ideal test, 66
Immunoglobulin G (IgG), 19
Immunoglobulin M (IgM), 19
immunological antibodies, 19
immunology, 9–12
    and genetics, 60–61
indices review, 71–72
innate maternal reducing systems,
    37–38

insulin resistance syndrome, 51
integrins, 70
intercellular matrix, 25
intercurrent eclampsia, 138
intrauterine growth restriction
    (IUGR), 16, 25, 85, 138
Iranian study, 54
isometric exercise test, 67
ISSHP classification, 127
IUGR (intrauterine growth
    restriction), 16, 25, 85, 138

K

kallikrein, 68

L

labetalol, 137
labour induction
    Bishop score for, **145**
    in eclampsia, 138
    Foley catheters in, 146
    methods of, 146
    in PIH, 137–138, 144
    in pregnancy, 138–139
    in severe pre-eclampsi, 138
    trachleodynamics in, 144–145
LDL, *see* low-density lipoprotein
    (LDL)
leucocytes, 68
lipid, 28, **52**, 53
    peroxidation, 32
    peroxides, 25–28
    transition metals in, 34–35
lipid peroxyl radical (LOO⁺), 34
lipoprotein molecules, 26
liver
    HELLP syndrome, 110
    pathological changes, 109–110
low-density lipoprotein (LDL), 26,
    26, 42
    phenotype, 31–32
lucid interval, 137
lysophosphotidyl choline, 46–47

M

malignancies, 83
malondialdehyde (MDA), 32–33
mammalian studies, 59

management goals, 133
MAP (mean arterial pressure), 67, 128
masked hypertension, 127
maternal weight gain in pregnancy, 67
MCA (middle cerebral artery) flow, 139, *141*, *142*
MDA (malondialdehyde), 32–33
mean arterial pressure (MAP), 67, 128
mean platelet volume (MPV), 69
membranous glomerulonephritis, 120
metabolic syndrome, 51, **52**
    diagnosis, 54
    and hypertension, 51–52
    and pre-eclampsia, 54
metallothionein, 20
methyl ergometrine, 147
microalbuminuria, 67
microscopy, 119–121
middle cerebral artery (MCA) flow, 139, *141*, *142*
mid-trimester blood pressure, 66–67
MOM (multiple of median), 71
mono therapy *versus* multi-drug therapy, 136–137
mouse model, 61
MPV (mean platelet volume), 69
multigravida, 145
multiple of median (MOM), 71
multiple tests, 65

N

National Health Service (NHS), 72
NDI (notch depth index), 74–75, *75*
negative and positive tests, clinical bearings, 66
neonatologist involvement, 144
neutrons, 23
neutrophil activation, 39
NHS (National Health Service), 72
nifedipine, 135–137
nitric oxide (NO), 41
nitric oxide synthase (NOS), 41
non-diseased states, 38
nonsteroidal anti-inflammatory drug (NSAID), 89
notch depth index (NDI), 74–75, *75*

O

obstetric vasculopathy, 4–5, 96
oedema, 129
oedematous lesions, 96
ophthalmic system, 113–114
oscillatory pressure, 100–101, *101*
oxidative stress, 23
    agents of, 25–28
    vascular endothelium and, 38–39

P

PAH (pregnancy-associated hypertension), 122–123
paradoxical phenomenon, 46
pathological lesions, 95–96
pathophysiology, 27
peripheral vascular resistance, 101
PGE2, 145–146
physiological stress, 46
PI (pulsatility index), 71
PIH, *see* pregnancy-induced hypertension (PIH)
placental atherosis, 42
placental growth hormone, 29
placental lipid peroxidation, 32–34
placental vasculopathy, 4
placentation, 10
platelets
    activation, 68–69
    activation and thromboxane A_2 production, 105–106
    competence alteration, concept of, 105
policeman-to-riot model, 43–44, 69
posterior leukoencephalopathy syndrome, 96
postpartum haemorrhage (PPH), 147
powerhouse reductant, 43–44
pre-eclampsia, 4, 127
    aspects, 3–4
    diagnosis and alert surveillance, 133–134
    exercise and prevention of, 45–46
    genetics roles in, 57–58, *58*
    genetic studies in, 58–59
    management on hospitalization, 134–139

normal pregnancy, lipid metabolism in, 28–31
    pregnancies, 104–105
    quality of tests, 65–66
    severity grades, 129
    tests for prediction in, 65
    types of, 9–10
pre-eclamptic toxaemia, 20
pregnancy-associated hypertension (PAH), 122–123
pregnancy-induced hypertension (PIH), 67
    caesarean section in, 146–147
    labour induction in, 137–138, 144
procoagulants, 103
    molecules, 17–18
propulsive pressure, 100–101, *101*
prostaglandins, 16–17, 145–146
proteins, 122
    and amino acids, 53
    thiol-disulphide oxidoreductases, 38
proteinuria, 127–129, 134
protons, 23
pulmonary oedema, 148
pulsatility index (PI), 71

R

reactive oxygen species (ROS), 23, 31
Reaven syndrome, 51
receiver operating curve (ROC), 65
recurrent and unilateral, visual alterations, 114
reducing systems
    ideal, 45
    inconsistency of, 45
    limitations, 44–45
    mechanism, *25*
renal failure, 148
    complicating pre-eclampsia, 118–119
renal function alterations, 121–122
renal glomerular capillary endotheliosis, 16
renal system, 117
    changes in pregnancy, 117
    function alterations in pre-eclampsia, 121–122
    lesions, 119

renal system (*Continued*)
  microscopy, 119–121
  pathognomonic, 119
  vulnerability of, 117–118
renin-angiotensin system, 122–123
reperfusion, 35–37, *36*
resistance index (RI), 71
ROC (receiver operating curve), 65
ROS (reactive oxygen species),
    23, 31

S

salt restriction, 85
Screening Programme for
    Pre-Eclampsia (SPREE), 72
SFH (symphysis-fundal height), 139
SLE (systemic lupus
    erythematosus), 4
Smith-Lemli-Opitz syndrome, 30
SOD (superoxide dismutase), 33
sodium nitroprusside, 135
SPREE (Screening Programme for
    Pre-Eclampsia), 72
stem cells, 84
stroke volume and heart rate, 99
sublethal injuries, 17
superoxide dismutase (SOD), 33
symphysis-fundal height (SFH), 139
syncytiotrophoblasts, 9–10
  microvesicles, 77
syndrome X, 51
systemic lupus erythematosus
    (SLE), 4

T

tests types, 66
thrombocytopenia, 103
thromboxane-prostacyclin balance,
    37, *106*
TMA (Trombotic
    Microangiopathies), 120
TNF-α (Tumor Necrosis Factor
    Alpha), 19
toxins, 20
trace elements and
    micronutrients, 87
Trombotic Microangiopathies
    (TMA), 120
trophoblastic invasion, inefficient
    second wave, 39–40
Tumor Necrosis Factor Alpha
    (TNF-α), 19
two-stage pregnancy, 10

U

UGKO (uterine gland knockout),
    11–12
ultra-low-density lipoprotein
    (ULDL), 26
ultrasonography, 71
umbilical artery flow, 139, *141*, *143*
unadulterated VLDLs, 30
uric acid, 43, 69
  policeman-to-riot model,
    43–44
urinary calcium, 68

urinary tests
  calcium-to-creatinine ratio, 68
  kallikrein, 68
  microalbuminuria, 67
  urinary calcium, 68
uterine gland knockout (UGKO),
    11–12
uterine glands and placentation,
    10–12
uterine milk, 11

V

vascular bed, 15, *15*
vascular endothelial growth
    factors (VEGFs), 18,
    40, 40–41
vascular endothelium, 38–39
vascular permeability factor, 18
vascular tone, 15
vasospasm, 16, 25, 28, 46, 121
VEGFs (vascular endothelial
    growth factors), 18, **40**,
    40–41
veins, 15, *15*
venous system, changes in, 101
venules, 15, *15*
very-low-density lipoprotein
    (VLDL), 26, *26*, 53
von Willebrand Factor (VWF), 18

W

white-coat hypertension, 127